Contents

2nd edition
High-Yield Histology

2nd edition
High-Yield Histology

Ronald W. Dudek, Ph.D.

Full Professor

Department of Anatomy and Cell Biology

East Carolina University School of Medicine

Greenville, North Carolina

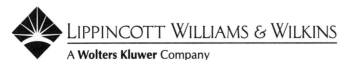

LIPPINCOTT WILLIAMS & WILKINS

A **Wolters Kluwer** Company

Philadelphia · Baltimore · New York · London
Buenos Aires · Hong Kong · Sydney · Tokyo

Editor: Elizabeth Nieginski
Development Editor: Donna Siegfried
Managing Editor: Marette D. Magargle-Smith
Marketing Manager: Aimee Sirmon

351 West Camden Street
Baltimore, Maryland 21201-2436 USA

530 Walnut Street
Philadelphia, Pennsylvania 19106 USA

Printed in the United States of America

Library of Congress Cataloging-in-Publication Data

Dudek, Ronald W., 1950–
    High-yield histology / Ronald W. Dudek.—2nd ed.
        p. ; cm.
    Includes index.
    ISBN 0-683-72134-2
    1. Histology—Examinations, questions, etc. 2. Histology—Outlines, syllabi, etc.
 I. Title.
    [DNLM: 1. Histology—Examination Questions. 2. Histology—Outlines. QS 518.2
D845h 2000]
QM554 .D83 2000
611'.018'076—dc21   99-057932

To purchase additional copies of this book, call our customer service department at **(800) 638-3030** or fax orders to **(301) 824-7390.** International customers should call **(301) 714-2324.**

00 01 02 03

1 2 3 4 5 6 7 8 9 10

Dedication

I would like to dedicate this book to my mother, Lottie Dudek, who was born on November 11, 1918. Through the years, my mother raised her children, maintained a loving marriage, cared for her aging parents, and worked 40 hours per week. In 1990s parlance, society would describe such a person as a "liberated woman" or "supermom." I would like to acknowledge that my mother was a "supermom" 20 years before the word was fashionable. A son cannot repay a mother. My hope is that "I love you and thank you" will suffice.

Preface

The second edition of *High-Yield Histology* has been a pleasure to write. Following the publication of the first edition, I received many comments from readers and reviewers concerning how well the book met the stated goal of the *High-Yield* series, specifically, to provide uncomplicated, concise coverage of only those topics that are extremely relevant when one is preparing for the United States Medical Licensing Examination (USMLE). In preparing the second edition, I have responded to these comments.

This exercise has led to the development of an unusual type of histology book. As you may know, the questions on the USMLE cross traditional course boundaries, making it difficult to identify a question that is "strictly histology." Many USMLE questions fall into categories such as histopathology, histophysiology, and histobiochemistry. To this end, the second edition of *High-Yield Histology* reviews basic histologic concepts and then extends the discussion to relevant areas in pathology, physiology, and biochemistry. This makes *High-Yield Histology* a truly integrated review book that reflects the way histology is tested on the USMLE Step 1.

In addition, many students have commented that cell biology and blood topics have been well represented on the USMLE Step 1. To this end, I have expanded Chapter 1, "Cell Biology," and added a chapter (Chapter 9, "Blood").

High-Yield Histology, 2nd edition; *High-Yield Embryology*, *High-Yield Gross Anatomy*, and *High-Yield Molecular Biology* comprise my contribution to the *High-Yield* series. I would appreciate any comments or suggestions concerning any of these review books, especially after you have taken the USMLE Step 1. You may contact me at dudek@brody.med.ecu.edu.

1
Cell Biology

I. NUCLEAR STRUCTURES

A. Nuclear envelope

1. The inner membrane is associated with a network of **intermediate filaments (lamins A, B, C)** called the **nuclear lamina,** which plays a role in the re-assembly of the nuclear envelope during telophase of mitosis. The outer membrane is studded with ribosomes and is continuous with the rough endoplasmic reticulum (rER).

2. The inner and outer membranes are separated by a **perinuclear cisterna.**

3. The **nuclear pore complex** consists of many different proteins arranged in octagonal symmetry with a central channel. The nuclear pore complex allows passage of molecules between the nucleus and cytoplasm (Table 1-1).

B. **Chromatin** is double-helical DNA associated with histones and nonhistone proteins.

1. **Heterochromatin** is **condensed** chromatin and is **transcriptionally inactive.** In electron micrographs, heterochromatin is electron dense. An example of heterochromatin is the **Barr body,** which is found in female cells and represents the inactive X chromosome.

2. **Euchromatin** is **dispersed** chromatin and is **transcriptionally active.**

3. A **nucleosome** consists of **DNA** coiled around **histones H2A, H2B, H3, and H4,** forming an 11-nm-diameter chromatin fiber. A nucleosome that has a "beads-on-a-string" appearance is the **basic unit of chromatin packaging.** These 11-nm chromatin fibers can be packaged together into 30-nm chromatin fibers by histone H1.

C. **Chromosomes** contain some specialized nucleotide sequences.

1. **Centromeres** are nucleotide sequences that mark the **primary constriction** along the chromosome. Protein complexes called **kinetochores** assemble at the centromere and bind microtubules of the mitotic spindle during mitosis.

2. **Telomeres** are nucleotide sequences (GGGTTA) located at the end of a chromosome that allow replication of DNA to its full length using the enzyme called **telomerase.**

3. The **replication origin** is a nucleotide sequence that serves as an origination site of chromosome replication. Human chromosomes contain numerous replication origins to ensure rapid replication. In humans, **DNA polymerase α and δ** catalyze DNA replication. Other DNA polymerases exist within the cell; namely **DNA**

Table 1-1
Molecular Transport Between Nucleus and Cytoplasm

	Direction of Movement	Mechanism
Ions Small molecules (< 5000 d) Proteins (< 60,000 d)	Nucleus → cytoplasm Nucleus ← cytoplasm	Passive transport (diffusion) No ATP hydrolysis
mRNA tRNA rRNA	Nucleus → cytoplasm	Active transport Requires ATP hydrolysis Requires binding of RNA to proteins with a signal sequence of 4–8 amino acids for recognition by the nuclear pore complex
Proteins (> 60,000 d) such as nucleoplasmin, steroid receptors, DNA and RNA polymerases, gene regulatory proteins, RNA-processing proteins	Nucleus ← cytoplasm	Active transport Requires ATP hydrolysis Requires a signal sequence of 4–8 amino acids for recognition by the nuclear pore complex

ATP = adenosine triphosphate; mRNA = messenger RNA; rRNA = ribosomal RNA; tRNA = transfer RNA.

polymerase **β and ε**, which catalyze DNA repair, and **DNA polymerase γ,** which catalyzes mitochondrial DNA replication.

D. The **nucleolus** consists of portions of five pairs of chromosomes (i.e., 13, 14, 15, 21, and 22) that contain genes that code for **ribosomal RNA (rRNA).** In humans, **RNA polymerase I** catalyzes the formation of rRNA. Other RNA polymerases exist within the cell; namely **RNA polymerase II,** which catalyzes the formation of messenger RNA (mRNA), and **RNA polymerase III,** which catalyzes the formation of transfer RNA (tRNA). By electron microscopy, three regions of the nucleolus can be distinguished.

1. The **fibrillar center** is pale-staining and contains transcriptionally inactive DNA.

2. The **dense fibrillar component** contains rRNA in the process of being synthesized.

3. The **granular component** contains rRNA bound to ribosomal proteins beginning to mature into ribosomes.

II. CYTOPLASM contains **enzymes** for glycolysis, fatty acid synthesis (i.e., fatty acid synthase), three reactions of the urea cycle (using argininosuccinate synthetase, argininosuccinate lyase, and arginase), glycogen synthesis and degradation, and protein synthesis, as well as **intermediates of metabolism** and many **cofactors.**

III. CYTOPLASMIC STRUCTURES

A. Ribosomes

1. Ribosomes consist of **40S (small)** and **60S (large) subunits** containing rRNA and various proteins (Table 1-2).

2. They are the sites where **translation of mRNA** into an amino acid sequence (i.e., protein synthesis) occurs.

3. Ribosomes may cluster along a strand of mRNA to form a **polyribosome** (or

Table 1-2
Ribosomal Subunits

Subunit	rRNA Type	Number of Proteins	Functions
40S	18S	$\cong 33$	Has binding sites for mRNA and tRNA Binds to mRNA and finds the start codon AUG
60S	5S, 5.8S, 28S	$\cong 49$	Binds to the 40S subunit after 40S subunit finds the start codon AUG Has peptidyl transferase activity

rRNA = ribosomal RNA; mRNA = messenger RNA; tRNA = transfer RNA.

polysome) that is involved in the **synthesis of cytoplasmic proteins** (e.g., actin, hemoglobulin).

4. They may be directed to the endoplasmic reticulum to form rER if the nascent protein contains a hydrophobic **signal sequence** at its amino terminal end, which is cleaved in the rER lumen by **signal peptidase.**

B. rER. This membranous organelle contains ribosomes attached to its cytoplasmic surface by the binding of **ribophorin I and II** to the **ribosomal 60S subunit.**

1. It is the site of **synthesis of secretory proteins** (e.g., insulin), **cell membrane proteins** (e.g., receptors), and **lysosomal enzymes.**

2. It is the site of **co-translational modification of proteins:**
   a. **N-linked glycosylation** (addition of sugars to asparagine begins in the rER and is completed in the Golgi complex)
   b. **Hydroxylation** of proline and lysine during collagen synthesis
   c. **Cleavage** of the signal sequence
   d. **Folding** of the nascent protein into three-dimensional configuration
   e. **Association** of protein subunits into multimeric complex

C. **Smooth endoplasmic reticulum (sER)** is a membranous organelle that contains no ribosomes. It is involved in:

1. **Synthesis of membrane phospholipids** (phosphatidylcholine, sphingomyelin, phosphatidylserine, phosphatidylthanolamine), cholesterol, and ceramide

2. **Synthesis of steroid hormones** in testes, ovary, adrenal cortex, and placenta

3. **Drug detoxification using cytochrome P$_{450}$,** which is a family of heme proteins (also called **mixed-function oxidase system**) that participates in hydroxylation of barbiturates, phenytoin, or benzopyrene (a carcinogen found in cigarette smoke), makes them more soluble in water, and allows excretion into the urine
   a. Activation of cytochrome P$_{450}$ by one agent enhances the detoxification of other agents, which has clinical implications.
   b. In **chronic alcoholics** or **newborns,** large amounts of anesthesia agents are needed (which may be dangerous) because cytochrome P$_{450}$ has been activated by detoxifying either alcohol or breakdown products of fetal hemoglobulin, respectively.

4. Fatty acid elongation

5. **Calcium fluxes** associated with muscle contraction

D. **Golgi complexes** are stacks of membranous cisternae with a *cis*-face (convex) that receives vesicles of newly synthesized proteins from the rER and a **trans-face** (concave) that releases condensing vacuoles of posttranslationally modified proteins.

1. It is the site of **posttranslational modification of proteins,** such as:
 a. **Completion of N-linked glycosylation** that began in the rER
 b. **O-linked glycosylation;** that is, addition of sugars to serine by the enzyme glycosyltransferase
 c. **Sulfation**
 d. **Phosphorylation** (phosphorylation of mannose forming **mannose-6-phosphate** occurs only in lysosomal enzymes)

2. It is involved in **protein sorting and packaging.**
 a. **Secretory proteins** (e.g., insulin) are packaged into clathrin-coated vesicles.
 b. **Cell membrane proteins** (e.g., receptors) are packaged into nonclathrin-coated vesicles.
 c. **Lysosomal enzymes** are packaged into clathrin-coated vesicles after phosphorylation of mannose.

3. It is involved in **membrane recycling.**

E. Mitochondria

1. **Function.** Mitochondria are involved in the production of acetyl coenzyme A (CoA), the tricarboxylic acid cycle, fatty acid β-oxidation, amino acid oxidation, and oxidative phosphorylation [which causes the **synthesis of adenosine triphosphate (ATP)** driven by electron transfer to oxygen].
 a. **Substrates** are metabolized in the mitochondrial matrix to produce **acetyl CoA,** which is **oxidized by the tricarboxylic acid cycle** to carbon dioxide.
 b. The energy released by this oxidation is captured by reduced nicotinamide adenine dinucleotide (NADH) and flavin adenine dinucleotide ($FADH_2$). NADH and $FADH_2$ are further oxidized, producing **hydrogen ions and electrons.**
 c. The electrons are transferred along the **electron transport chain,** which is accompanied by the outward pumping of hydrogen ions into the intermembrane space (**chemiosmotic theory**).
 d. The F_0 subunit of ATP synthase forms a transmembrane hydrogen ion pore so that hydrogen ions can flow from the intermembrane space into the matrix, where the F_1 subunit of ATP synthase catalyzes the reaction $ADP + P_i \rightarrow ATP$.

2. **Components and contents** are listed in Table 1-3.

3. **Clinical considerations**
 a. **Leder's hereditary optic neuropathy** is characterized by progressive optic nerve degeneration and is caused by a mitochondrial DNA mutation in the gene for **subunit 4 of the NADH dehydrogenase complex.** Mitochondrial diseases are **maternally inherited** and affect tissues that have a high requirement for ATP (e.g., nerve, muscle).
 b. **Myoclonic epileptic ragged red fiber disease** is characterized by progressive myoclonus (muscle jerking), dementia, and hearing loss. It is caused by a mitochondrial DNA mutation in the gene for **tRNA for lysine.**
 c. **Cyanide, carbon monoxide,** and **antimycin A** inhibit the electron transport chain and thus block ATP synthesis.
 d. **Oligomycin** and **venturicidin** are antibiotics that bind to ATP synthase and thus block ATP synthesis.

F. Lysosomes are membrane-bound organelles that contain lysosomal enzymes (also called **acid hydrolase enzymes**) including cathepsin B and L (proteases), nuclease, 5′-nucleoti-

Table 1-3

Components and Contents

Components	Contents
Outer membrane	Porin (a transport protein that increases permeability to metabolic sustrates)
Intermembrane space	Hydrogen ions
Inner membrane (folded into cristae)	Electron transport chain (NADH dehydrogenase, succinate dehydrogenase, ubiquinone-cytochrome c oxidoreductase, cytochrome oxidase)
	ATP synthase (found on elementary particles)
	ATP–ADP translocator (moves ADP into the matrix and ATP out of the matrix)
Matrix compartment	Tricarboxylic acid (TCA) cycle enzymes (except succinate dehydrogenase)
	Fatty acid β-oxidation enzymes
	Amino acid oxidation enzymes
	Pyruvate dehydrogenase complex
	Carbamoylphosphate synthetase I
	Ornithine transcarbamoylase (part of urea cycle)
	DNA, mRNA, tRNA, rRNA
	Granules containing calcium and magnesium ions

NADH = reduced nicotinamide adenine dinucleotide; mRNA = messenger RNA; rRNA = ribosomal RNA; tRNA = transfer RNA; ATP = adenosine triphosphate (ATP); ADP = adenosine diphosphate (ADP).

dase, β-galactosidase, β-glucuronidase, glycosidase, aryl sulfatase, lipase, esterase, and acid phosphatase that function at **pH 5.** Most lysosomes function intracellularly; however, some cells (e.g., neutrophils, osteoclasts) release their lysosomal contents extracellularly.

1. **Golgi hydrolase vesicles** bud from the Golgi complex and contain inactive acid hydrolase enzymes.

   a. Golgi hydrolase vesicles fuse with a **late endosome,** which contains an H^+-ATPase in its membrane that produces a pH 5 environment, which activates the acid hydrolases.

   b. A late endosome may fuse with a phagocytic vacuole forming a **phagolysosome,** which degrades material phagocytosed by the cell.

   c. A late endosome may fuse with an autophagic vacuole forming an **autophagolysosome,** which degrades cell organelles.

2. **Residual bodies** contain undigestible material and may accumulate within a cell as **lipofuscin pigment.**

3. **Clinical considerations.** There are a number of genetic diseases that involve mutations of genes for various lysosomal enzymes (acid hydrolases; Table 1-4).

G. **Peroxisomes** are membrane-bound organelles.

1. **Contents of peroxisomes** include:

   a. **Amino acid oxidase** and **hydroxyacid oxidase,** which produce **hydrogen peroxide (H_2O_2)**

   b. **Catalase** and **other peroxidases** that decompose hydrogen peroxide to water and oxygen ($H_2O_2 \rightarrow H_2O + O_2$)

   c. **Fatty acid β-oxidation enzymes** that oxidize long-chain fatty acids (> 20 carbons) to short-chain fatty acids, which are transferred to mitochondria for complete oxidation

2. **Clinical consideration. Adrenoleukodystrophy** is a genetic disease that involves

Table 1-4
Lysosomal Storage Diseases

Disease	Enzyme Involved	Major Accumulating Metabolite
Hurler's disease	L-iduronidase	Heparan sulfate Deramatan sulfate
Sanfilippo A	Heparan sulfamidase	Heparan sulfate
Tay-Sachs disease	Hexosaminidase A	GM_2 ganglioside
Gaucher's disease	β-glucosidase	Glucosylceramide
Niemann-Pick disease	Sphingomyelinase	Sphingomyelin
Pompe's disease	α-1, 4-Glucosidase (acid maltase)	Glycogen
I-cell disease	Phosphotransferase	Mucopolysaccharide
Krabbe's disease	β-galactosidase	Galactosylceramide

mutation of genes for various **peroxisomal enzymes** used in fatty acid β-oxidation that results in abnormal **accumulation of lipid** in the brain, spinal cord, and adrenal gland and leads to **dementia** and **adrenal failure.**

IV. CYTOSKELETON

   A.   Filamentous actin (F-actin)

   1. F-actin comprises microfilaments (6-nm diameter) arranged in a helix of polymerized **globular monomers of actin (G-actin).**

   2. It is in a constant state of polymerization and depolymerization.

   3. F-actin functions in exocytosis, endocytosis, cytokinesis, locomotion of cells forming lamellipodia, and movement of cell membrane proteins.

   4. **Cytochalasin** is a toxic fungal alkaloid that causes F-actin to depolymerize.

   5. **Phalloidin** is a toxic substance derived from the *Amanita* mushroom that binds to F-actin, thereby inhibiting polymerization/depolymerization.

   B.   Intermediate filaments (10-nm to 12-nm diameter)

   1. These function as the cytoplasmic link between the extracellular matrix, cytoplasm, and nucleus.

   2. Intermediate filaments demonstrate specificity (Table 1-5) for certain cell types/tumors, and therefore can be used as markers for pathologic analysis.

   C.   Microtubules are 25-nm-diameter tubules that consist of 13 circularly arranged proteins called **α and β tubulin.**

   1. They are in dynamic equilibrium with a cytoplasmic pool of α and β tubulin such that a polymerization end [**plus (+) end**] and a depolymerization end [**minus (−) end**] are present on each microtubule.

   2. Microtubules are always associated with **microtubule-associated proteins (MAPs).**
      a. **Kinesin** has ATPase activity for movement of vesicles along microtubules toward the plus end (**anterograde transport**).
      b. **Dynein** has ATPase activity for movement of vesicles along microtubules toward the minus end (**retrograde transport**).
      c. **Dynamin** has ATPase activity for elongation of nerve axons.

Table 1-5
Specifity of Intermediate Filaments for Cell Types or Tumors

Intermediate Filament	Cell or Tumor Specificity
Cytokeratin	Epithelial cells Epithelial tumors (e.g., squamous carcinoma, adenocarcinoma)
Vimentin	Endothelial cells, vascular smooth muscle, fibroblasts, chondroblasts, and macrophages Mesenchymal tumors (e.g., fibrosarcoma, liposarcoma, angiosarcoma, chondrosarcoma, osteosarcoma)
Desmin	Skeletal muscle, nonvascular smooth muscle Muscle tumors (e.g., rhabdomyosarcoma)
Neurofilament	Neurons Neuronal tumors
Glial fibrillar acidic protein (GFAP)	Astrocytes, oligodendroglia, microglia, Schwann cells, ependymal cells, and pituicytes Gliomatous tumors
Lamins A, B, C	Inner membrane of nuclear envelope

3. **Functions** of microtubules include maintaining cell shape (polarity), movement of chromosomes (karyokinesis), movement of secretory granules and neurosecretory vesicles, beating of cilia and flagella, and phagocytosis/lysosomal function.

4. The **microtubular organizing center** of the cell for the assembly of microtubules is called the **centrosome.** At the center of the centrosome are two hollow structures oriented perpendicular to each other called the **centriole.**

5. Clinical considerations
  a. **Chédiak-Higashi syndrome** is a genetic disease characterized by neutropenia and impaired phagocytosis of bacteria due to a **defect in microtubule polymerization** that **impairs lysosomal function** of leukocytes. Large abnormal lysosomes can be observed in the cytoplasm of leukocytes in people with this syndrome.
  b. **Colchicine** is an antimitotic agent that inhibits microtubule assembly.
  c. **Taxol** is an antimitotic agent that stabilizes microtubule movement.

V. CELL MEMBRANE. The cell membrane (8~ to 10~nm thick) appears in electron microscopy of osmium-fixed tissue as two electron-dense lines separated by an electron-lucent space. The electron-dense lines are due to the deposition of osmium on the hydrophilic heads of lipids. The electron-lucent space represents the hydrophobic tails of lipids.

A. The **lipid component** consists of four phospholipids: **phosphatidylcholine, sphingomyelin, phosphatidylethanolamine, and phosphatidylserine. Cholesterol and glycolipids** (e.g., ganglioside GM_1) also are present.

1. The lipids that constitute the lipid bilayer are **amphiphilic;** that is, they have a **hydrophilic (polar) head** and a **hydrophobic (nonpolar) tail.**

2. The lipid component exhibits **asymmetry** in which **phosphatidylcholine and sphingomyelin** are located in the outer leaflet; **phosphatidylethanolamine and phosphatidylserine** are located in the inner leaflet.

3. The lipid component exhibits **fluidity,** which means that the phospholipids diffuse laterally within the lipid bilayer.

    a. Fluidity is **increased** by increases in both **temperature** and **degree of unsaturation** of the fatty acid tails.

    b. Fluidity is **decreased** by increases in **cholesterol** content.

B. **The protein component**

    1. **Composition.** The protein component consists of peripheral and integral proteins.

        a. **Peripheral proteins** can be easily disassociated from the lipid bilayer by changes in **ionic strength or pH.**

        b. **Integral proteins** are difficult to disassociate from the lipid bilayer unless detergents [e.g., sodium dodecyl sulfate or **Triton X-100**] are used. **Transmembrane proteins** are integral proteins that span the lipid bilayer, exposing the protein to both the extracellular space and the cytoplasm. Many transmembrane proteins are now known to be receptor proteins.

    2. Receptor proteins

        a. **Ion channel-linked receptors** are proteins that include voltage-gated ion channels, mechanical-gated ion channels, and neurotransmitter-gated ion channels.

            (1) Neurotransmitter-gated ion channels are receptors that bind neurotransmitters and mediate ion movement.

            (2) Some important neurotransmitter-gated ion channels are the **nicotinic acetylcholine receptor, the 5-hydroxytryptamine serotonin receptor, the N-methyl-D-aspartate receptor, the γ-aminobutyric acid receptor, and the glycine receptor.**

        b. **G-protein–linked receptors** are proteins that span the cell membrane seven times and are linked to **trimeric GTP-binding proteins (called G proteins).** These receptors activate a chain of cellular events either through the cyclic adenosine monophosphate (cAMP) pathway or calcium ion (Ca^{2+}) pathway.

            (1) **The cAMP pathway** increases or decreases cAMP levels by stimulation or inhibition of adenylate cyclase, respectively.

            (2) **The calcium ion pathway** activates **phospholipase C,** which cleaves phosphatidylinositol biphosphate into inositol triphosphate (IP_3) and diacylglycerol (DAG).

                (a) **Inositol triphosphate** causes the release of calcium ions from the endoplasmic reticulum, which activates the enzyme **Ca^{2+}/calmodulin-dependent protein kinase (Cam-kinase).**

                (b) **Diacylglycerol** activates the enzyme **protein kinase C (PKC).** Some important G-protein–linked receptors are the **muscarinic acetylcholine receptor, the α- and β-adrenergic receptors, the dopamine receptor, and the glucagon receptor.**

        c. **Enzyme-linked receptors** are proteins that span the cell membrane one time and are linked to an enzyme (e.g., **tyrosine kinase**). When the appropriate signal binds to a receptor, its intrinsic tyrosine kinase autophosphorylates tyrosine residues within the receptor.

            (1) This activates a chain of cellular events that includes SH_2 (*src* [Roux sarcoma virus] homology) domain proteins, **Sos (son-of-sevenless protein), Ras protein** (a gene product of *ras* proto-oncogene), **Raf protein kinase,** and **mitogen-activated protein (MAP) kinase,** which eventually affects gene transcription within the nucleus.

            (2) Some important enzyme-linked receptors are the **insulin receptor, the epidermal growth factor (EGF) receptor, and the fibroblast growth factor (FGF) receptor.**

    3. The protein component exhibits **patching** or **capping,** which means that proteins diffuse laterally with the lipid bilayer.

4. The protein component is studied by electron microscopy (EM) using the **freeze-fracture technique,** whereby the lipid bilayer is cleaved between the inner and outer leaflets.

    a. The **P-face** is the outer surface of the inner leaflet and contains the majority of integral proteins, which are seen by EM as "bumps."

    b. The **E-face** is the inner surface of the outer leaflet and is seen by EM as a smooth surface with "pits."

5. The protein component is well characterized in **red blood cell (RBC) membranes** and includes the following proteins (Figure 1-1):

    a. **Spectrin** maintains the biconcave shape of the RBC. The tail ends of spectrin bind to **actin** and **band 4.1 protein.**

    b. **Ankyrin** attaches to **spectrin** and **band 3 protein.**

    c. **Band 3 protein** is an anion transporter that allows **bicarbonate ion** (HCO_3^-) to cross the RBC membrane in exchange for chloride ions (Cl^-).

    d. **Glycophorin** is the first transmembrane protein for which a complete amino acid sequence was determined. Its hydrophilic amino-terminal end is exposed to the extracellular space, its hydrophobic portion (22 amino acids long arranged in an α-helix) spans the lipid bilayer, and its hydrophilic carboxyl-terminal end is exposed to the cytoplasm.

C. **Clinical consideration. Familial hypercholesterolemia** is a genetic disease involving a mutation in the **low-density lipoprotein (LDL) receptor** in which patients have greatly elevated levels of serum cholesterol and suffer myocardial infarctions early in life. The mutation in the LDL receptor blocks a normal process called **receptor-mediated endocytosis,** which involves the following steps:

1. Circulating **serum LDL** binds to the **LDL receptor** located on the cell membrane, and the complex undergoes endocytosis as **clathrin-coated vesicles.**

2. The clathrin-coated vesicles fuse with cytoplasmic **early endosomes,** where LDL disassociates from the LDL receptor, and the LDL receptor is recycled to the cell membrane.

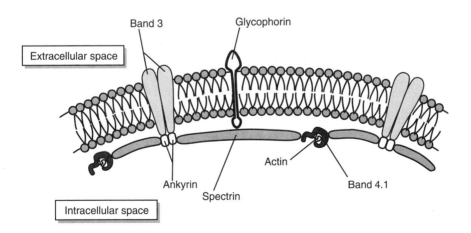

Figure 1-1. A schematic diagram of the red blood cell (RBC) membrane depicting the well-characterized protein component.

3. The early endosomes fuse with **late endosomes** containing active lysosomal enzymes that digest the LDL to **cholesterol.**

4. Cholesterol inhibits **3-hydroxy-3-methyglutaryl CoA reductase,** which suppresses de novo cholesterol synthesis, and therefore maintains normal levels of serum cholesterol.

VI. CELL CYCLE

A. Phases (Table 1-6)

B. Control factors of the cell cycle

Table 1-6
Phases of the Cell Cycle

	Phases	Cellular Events
	G_0 (gap)	Resting phase Cell cycle is suspended
	G_1 (gap) (5 hours)	RNA, protein, and organelle synthesis occurs. Cdk2–cyclin D and Cdk2–cyclin E form.
	G_1 Checkpoint	
Interphase	S (synthesis) (7 hours)	DNA synthesis occurs. RNA and histone synthesis occurs. Centrosome (MTOC) duplicates but remains together as a complex on one side of the nucleus.
	G_2 (gap) (3 hours)	ATP synthesis occurs. Cdk1-cyclin A and Cdk1-cyclin B form.
	G_2 Checkpoint	
	Prophase	Chromatin condenses to form well-defined chromosomes. Centrosomes (MTOC) move to opposite poles. Mitotic spindle (microtubules) forms between the centrosomes.
	Prometaphase	The nuclear envelope is disrupted. The nucleolus disappears. Kinetochores assemble at each centromere. Kinetochore, polar, and astral microtubules are apparent.
Mitosis **(M Phase)** (1 hour)	Metaphase	Chromosomes align at the metaphase plate. Cells can be arrested in this phase by microtubule inhibitors (e.g., colchicine). Cells can be isolated for karyotype analysis.
	Anaphase	Kinetochores separate, and chromosomes move to opposite poles.
	Telophase	Chromosomes decondense to form chromatin. The nuclear envelop re-forms. The nucleolus reappears.
	Cytokinesis	Cytoplasm divides by a process called cleavage. A cleavage furrow forms around the middle of the cell. A contractile ring consisting of actin and myosin forms at the cleavage furrow.

*Based on a 16-hour cell cycle.
MTOC = microtubular organizing center.

1. Cyclin-dependent protein kinase 1 and 2 (Cdk1 and Cdk2) induce cell cycle events by phosphorylation of target proteins. Cdk activity is controlled by cyclins.

2. **Cyclins** are produced by a family of related genes. Cyclins bind to Cdk and control the ability of Cdk to phosphorylate.
   a. **Cdk2–cyclin D** and **Cdk2–cyclin E** form during G_1 and mediate the transition from G_1 phase to the S phase at the G_1 **checkpoint.**
   b. **Cdk1–cyclin A** and **Cdk1–cyclin B** form during G_2 and mediate the transition from G_2 phase to the M phase at the G_2 **checkpoint.**

3. **Retinoblastoma (Rb) protein** is coded for by an **anti-oncogene** (or **tumor suppressor gene**). Rb protein binds to gene regulatory proteins such that there is no expression of target genes that stimulate the cell cycle. Therefore, the Rb protein causes **suppression of the cell cycle.** Mutations in the Rb anti-oncogene cause **retinoblastoma tumor,** which occurs in childhood and develops from precursor cells in the immature retina.

4. **The p53 zinc finger protein** is coded for by an **anti-oncogene** (or **tumor suppressor gene**). p53 causes expression of target genes whose gene products suppress the cell cycle at G_1 by **inhibiting Cdk2–cyclin D and Cdk2–cyclin E.** Therefore, p53 causes **suppression of the cell cycle.** Mutations in the p53 anti-oncogene play a role in **Li-Fraumeni syndrome,** which is an inherited susceptibility to a variety of cancers in which 50% of the affected individuals develop cancer by age 30 and 90% by age 70.

5. **The BRCA (breast cancer) zinc finger protein** is coded for by an **anti-oncogene** (or **tumor suppressor gene**). BRCA causes **suppression of the cell cycle.** Mutations in the BRCA anti-oncogene play a role in **breast and ovarian cancer.**

VII. APOPTOSIS is a distinctive form of cell death that is characterized by **chromatin clumping** into a distinct crescent pattern along the inner margins of the nuclear envelope and then into a dense body. The chromatin is eventually cleaved by a specific endonuclease into DNA fragments that generate a distinctive **180-bp ladder** that is pathognomonic of apoptotic cell death. The *bcl-2 gene* encodes an intracellular inhibitor of apoptosis. Apoptosis occurs in hormone-dependent involution of cells during the menstrual cycle, embryogenesis, toxin-induced injury (e.g., diphtheria), viral cell death (e.g., Councilman bodies in yellow fever), and cell death via cytotoxic T cells or other immune cells. Apoptosis does not elicit an inflammatory response.

VIII. CELL INCLUSIONS

A. **Lipofuscin** is a yellow-brown "wear and tear" pigment found predominately in residual bodies, which are the end point of lysosomal digestion.

   1. It is composed of **phospholipids complexed with proteins,** suggesting that it is derived from the lysosomal digestion of cellular membranes.

   2. Lipofuscin is a telltale sign of **free radical damage** and is found prominently within hepatocytes, skeletal muscle cells, and nerve cells of elderly people or patients with severe malnutrition.

B. **Hemosiderin** is a golden brown **hemoglobin-derived** pigment consisting of **iron.**

   1. Iron is **absorbed** mainly by **surface absorptive cells** within the **duodenum,** transported in the plasma by a protein called **transferrin,** and is normally stored in cells as **ferritin,** which is a protein–iron complex.

   2. Small amounts of ferritin normally circulate in the plasma, making **plasma ferritin** a good indicator of the adequacy of **body iron stores.**

   a. In **iron deficiency,** serum ferritin is less than 12 μg/L.
   b. In **iron overload,** serum ferritin approaches 5000 μg/L.
      (1) Also during iron overload, intracellular ferritin undergoes **lysosomal degradation,** in which the ferritin protein is degraded and the **iron aggregates** within the cell as hemosiderin in a condition called **hemosiderosis.**
      (2) Hemosiderosis can be observed in patients with **increased absorption of dietary iron, impaired utilization of iron, hemolytic anemias,** and **blood transfusions.**

C. Glycogen is the **storage form of glucose** and is composed of glucose units linked by **α-1,4 glycosidic bonds.** Glycogen synthesis is catalyzed by **glycogen synthase.** Glycogen degradation is catalyzed by **glycogen phosphorylase.** Liver hepatocytes and skeletal muscle cells contain the largest glycogen stores, but the function of glycogen differs widely.

   1. **Liver glycogen** functions in the **maintenance of blood glucose levels.**
      a. **Synthesis.** Liver glycogen is synthesized (using glycogen synthase) during a high-carbohydrate meal due to **hyperglycemia** and an **increase in the insulin:glucagon ratio.**
      b. **Degradation.** Liver glycogen is degraded (using liver glycogen phosphorylase isoenzyme) during **hypoglycemia** (e.g., fasting), **exercise,** or other **stressful situations** due to a **decrease in the insulin:glucagon ratio** and the **secretion of epinephrine** from the adrenal medulla, which binds to α- and β-adrenergic receptors on the hepatocyte.
         (1) Liver glycogen is degraded to **glucose-6-phosphate,** which is catalyzed to free glucose by the enzyme glucose-6-phosphatase.
         (2) **Glucose-6-phosphatase** is found only in the liver and kidney.

   2. **Skeletal muscle glycogen** functions in the **formation of ATP** through **glycolysis.**
      a. **Synthesis.** Skeletal muscle glycogen is synthesized (using glycogen synthase) during a high-carbohydrate meal due to **hyperglycemia** and an **increase in the insulin:glucagon ratio.**
      b. **Degradation.** Skeletal muscle glycogen is degraded (using muscle glycogen phosphorylase isoenzyme) during **exercise or stressful situations** due to a **decrease in ATP, calcium released during contraction,** and **secretion of epinephrine** from the adrenal medulla, which binds to α- and β-adrenergic receptors on the skeletal muscle cell.
         (1) Skeletal muscle glycogen is degraded to **glucose-6-phosphate,** which enters glycolysis to produce ATP.
         (2) The absence of **glucose-6-phosphatase** enzyme in skeletal muscle prevents the degradation of glycogen to free glucose.

   3. **Glycogen storage diseases** are genetic diseases that involve mutations in one of the enzymes of glycogen synthesis or degradation.
      a. **Von Gierke disease (type 1 glycogenosis)** results from a deficiency in the enzyme **glucose-6-phosphatase,** causing an **enlarged liver** and **severe hypoglycemia.**
      b. **McArdle disease (type V glycogenosis)** results from a deficiency in the enzyme muscle **glycogen phosphorylase,** causing **exercise-induced muscle pain and cramps.**

IX. SELECTED PHOTOMICROGRAPHS

A. Nuclear envelope and nuclear pore complex (Figure 1-2; see I A)

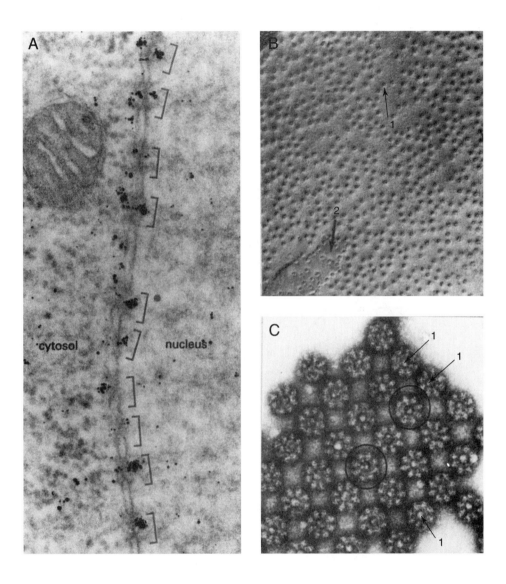

Figure 1-2. (A) Electron micrograph of nucleoplasmin labeled with colloidal gold particles. Nucleoplasmin is a large protein synthesized in the cytoplasm and transported into the nucleus. *Brackets* denote a nuclear pore complex. Note that the gold particles are localized specifically at the nuclear pore complex as nucleoplasmin moves from the cytoplasm to the nucleus. (Reproduced with permission from Feldherr C, Kallenbach E, Schultz N: *J Cell Biol* 99:2216, 1984 by copyright permission of the The Rockefeller University Press.) (B) A freeze-fracture replica of the nuclear envelope is shown. Note the nuclear pore complex (*arrow 1*). In addition, the outer membrane of the nuclear envelope has been stripped away (*arrow 2*), exposing the perinuclear cisterna. (Reproduced with permission from Stafstrom J, Stahelin L: *J Cell Biol* 98:699, 1984 by copyright permission of the Rockefeller University Press.) (C) Electron micrograph of octagonal protein complexes isolated from the nuclear envelope and negatively stained. Note the nuclear pore complex (*circles*) and a central channel or central pore (*arrow 1*). (Reproduced with permission from Unwin P: *J Cell Biol* 93:63, 1982 by copyright permission of The Rockefeller University Press.)

B. Chromatin (exons and introns) and nucleosomes (Figure 1-3; see I B)

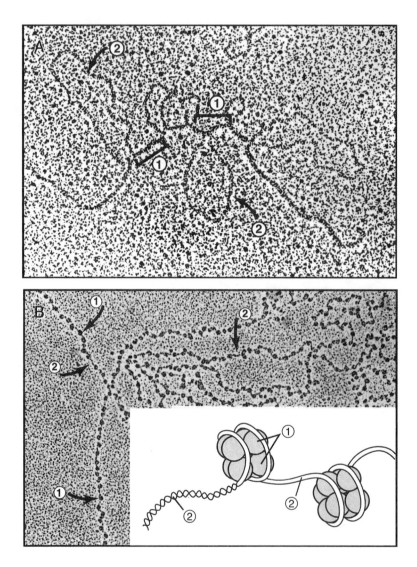

Figure 1-3. (A) Electron micrograph of DNA containing the gene for ovalbumin hybridized with ovalbumin messenger RNA (mRNA). Linear regions of the gene (*bracket 1*) that hybridize to mRNA are called **exons** because the processed mRNA "exits" the nucleus into the cytoplasm to participate in translation. Looped regions of the gene (*arrow 2*) that do not hybridize to mRNA are called **introns.** (Reprinted with permission from Chambon P: *Sci Am* 244:60, 1981.) (B) Electron micrograph of DNA isolated and subjected to treatments that unfold its native structure. This "beads-on-a-string" appearance is the basic unit of chromatin packing called a **nucleosome.** The globular structure ("bead"; *arrow 1*) is a histone octamer that is composed of specific proteins (H2A, H2B, H3, and H4). The linear structure ("string"; *arrow 2*) is DNA. (Reprinted with permission from McKnight S, Miller OL: *Cell* 8:305, 1976.) *Inset:* A diagram of a nucleosome depicting the histone octamer (*arrow 1*) and DNA (*arrow 2*).

C. Nucleus, rER, sER, Golgi complex, and mitochondria (Figure 1-4; see III B–E)

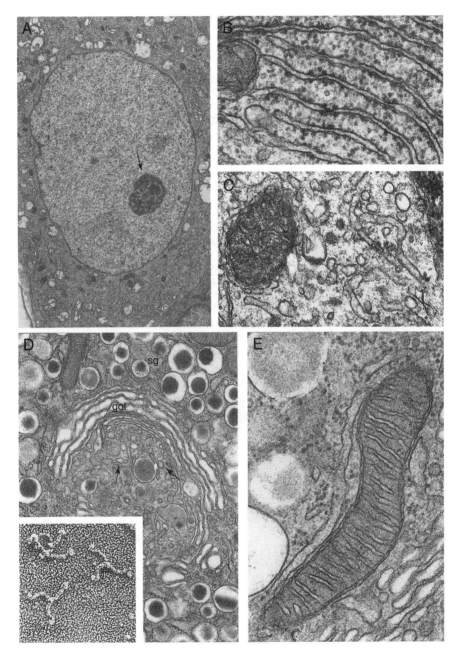

Figure 1-4. Electron micrographs of various cell organelles. (A) Nucleus containing predominately euchromatin and a conspicuous nucleolus (*arrow*). (B) Rough endoplasmic reticulum (rER), which shows membrane cisternae that are dotted with ribosomes. (C) Smooth endoplasmic reticulum (sER). (D) Golgi (*gol*) complex surrounded by many secretory granules (*sg*) and clathrin-coated vesicles (*arrows*) budding from the trans-face (concave). *Inset:* Isolated clathrin showing a distinctive three-legged structure called a **triskelion.** (E) Mitochondria and cristae.

D. Protein-secreting cell (Figure 1-5)

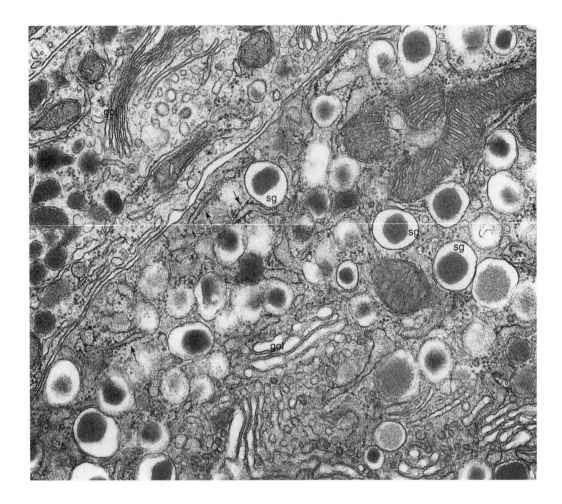

Figure 1-5. Electron micrograph of a protein-secreting cell containing prominent rough endoplasmic reticulum (rER; *arrows*), Golgi (*gol*) complex, and secretory granules (*sg*), which are conspicuous organelles in protein-secreting cells. (Courtesy of Dr. Jack Brinn, East Carolina University School of Medicine.)

E. **Steroid-secreting cell** (Figure 1-6)

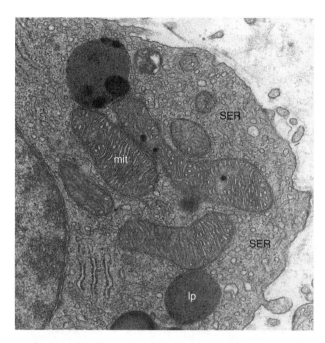

Figure 1-6.   Electron micrograph of a steroid-secreting cell containing prominent smooth endoplasmic reticulum (sER), mitochondria with tubular cristae (mit), and lipid droplets (lp), which are conspicuous organelles in steroid-secreting cells. (Courtesy of Dr. Jack Brinn, East Carolina University School of Medicine.)

F. **Apoptosis** (Figure 1-7; see VII)

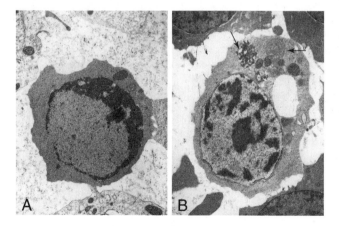

Figure 1-7.   (A, B) Electron micrographs of human T cells treated with a lipid hydroperoxide that is toxic to cells and induces cell death. Note the chromatin clumping and mitochondrial changes (*arrows in B*). These cells are in the process of cell death, called apoptosis. The chromatin of an apoptotic cell condenses into a distinctive crescent-shaped pattern (see A) along the inner margins of the nuclear envelope and then into a dense body that eventually breaks into fragments (see B). During these morphologic changes, the DNA is cleaved to generate a distinctive 180-bp ladder, which is pathognomonic of apoptotic cell death. The *bcl-2* gene has been cloned and encodes for an intracellular inhibitor of apoptosis. (Courtesy of D. Whitehead, East Carolina University School of Medicine.)

G. Transformation of normal cell to cancer cell (Figure 1-8)

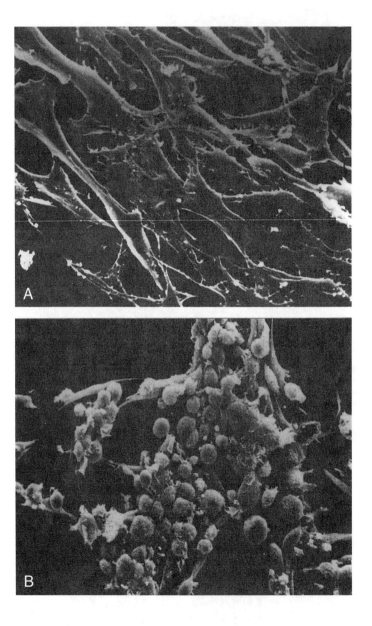

Figure 1-8.   Scanning electron micrographs of fibroblasts in culture infected with Roux sarcoma virus (src) that carries a temperature-sensitive mutation in the gene responsible for transformation (*v-src* oncogene). (A) When cultured at 39°C, the oncogene product is inactive, and these cells appear normal. Normal fibroblasts in nonconfluent cultures appear flat, attach firmly to substratum, spread under tension by the activity of lamellipodia and filopodia (locomotion organelles), and demonstrate contact inhibition of locomotion and cell division when the cells contact each other. (B) When cultured at 34°C, the oncogene product is active, and the cells are transformed, or "cancerous." Transformed fibroblasts in culture appear round, attach poorly to substratum, are capable of cell division to an unusually high density, do not demonstrate contact inhibition of locomotion or cell division, and cause tumors when injected into susceptible animals. (Courtesy of Dr. G. S. Martin, University of California at Berkeley.)

2
Epithelium

I. **INTRODUCTION.** Epithelium is a tissue that **covers the body surface, lines body cavities** (e.g., peritoneal, pleural), **lines tubules** (e.g., gastrointestinal tract, blood vessels, kidney tubules), and **forms glands** (e.g., exocrine, endocrine). Epithelium is **avascular** and has a **high regeneration capacity** ranging from a **few days** (e.g., epithelium lining small intestine) to **1 month** (e.g., epidermis of the skin).

II. **CLASSIFICATION** (Table 2-1)

III. **POLARITY** of an epithelial cell is made evident by specializations that are found in various regions of the cell (Figure 2-1).

A. **The apical region**

1. **Microvilli** contain a core of **actin** filaments that are anchored to the **terminal web.** The actin filaments are cross-linked by **villin.** Microvilli of intestinal epithelium are coated with a **glycocalyx** that consists of **terminal oligosaccharides of integral membrane proteins.** The glycocalyx has enzymatic activity involved in carbohydrate digestion.

2. **Stereocilia** are long microvilli found on **epididymal epithelium** and **hair cells of the inner ear.**

3. **Cilia** are motile cell processes that contain a core of microtubules (α and β tubulin) called the **axoneme.** The axoneme consists of nine doublet microtubules uniformly spaced around two central microtubules (**9 + 2 arrangement**). **Nexin** connects the nine doublet microtubules. Each doublet has **short arms** that consist of **dynein ATPase,** which splits ATP to provide energy for cilia movement. At the base of each cilium is a **basal body** that consists of nine triplet microtubules and no central microtubules (**9 + 0 arrangement**).

B. **The lateral region**

1. **The zonula occludens (or tight junction)** extends around the **entire perimeter** of the cell.
   a. The outer leaflets of the cell membrane of the two adjoining cells **fuse** at various points.
   b. The zonula occludens prevents or retards the diffusion of material across an epithelium via the **paracellular pathway** (i.e., through the intercellular space). Various epithelia have been classified either as "tight" or "leaky" based on the **permeability** of the zonula occludens.
   c. The zonula occludens can be rapidly formed and disassembled (e.g., **during leukocyte migration across endothelium**).

Table 2-1
Classification of Epithelium

Type of Epithelium	Location in Body
Simple squamous	**Type I pneumocytes** of alveoli, parietal layer of Bowman's capsule, **endothelium** of blood and lymph vessels, **mesothelium** of body cavities, **corneal endothelium**
Simple cuboidal	Lining of respiratory bronchioles, thyroid **follicular cells, germinal epithelium** of ovary, lens of eye, **pigment epithelium** of retina, **ependymal cells** of choroid plexus
Simple columnar	Lining of pulmonary bronchioles, lining of gastrointestinal tract, lining of anal canal **above anal valves,** lining of uterus and uterine tubes, lining of large excretory ducts of glands
Stratified squamous	**Epidermis** of skin, lining of oral cavity and esophagus, lining of anal canal **below anal valves,** lining of vagina, **corneal epithelium,** lining of female urethra, lining of **fossa navicularis** of the penile urethra
Stratified columnar	Lining of prostatic, membranous, and penile urethra up to fossa navicularis
Psudostratified columnar	Lining of trachea and primary bronchi; lining of efferent ductules, epididymis, and ductus deferens
Transitional	Lining of renal calyces, renal pelvis, ureters, and urinary bladder

2. **The zonula adherens** extends around the **entire perimeter** of the cell.
   a. The cell membranes of the two adjoining cells are separated by an intercellular space filled with an amorphous material.
   b. There is a dense area on the cytoplasmic side of each cell that consists of **actin filaments,** which are linked by **a-actinin** and **vinculin** to a transmembrane protein called **E-cadherin** [or adherens cell adhesion molecule (A-CAM)].

3. **The macula adherens (desmosome)** occurs at **small discrete sites.**
   a. The cell membranes of the two adjoining cells are separated by an intercellular space filled with a **thin dense line** of material. An **attachment plaque** on the cytoplasmic side of each cell anchors **tonofilaments.**
   b. Several protein components of the desmosome have been identified:
      (1) **Desmoglein I and desmocollin I and II** are calcium-binding proteins that mediate calcium-dependent cell adhesion.
      (2) **Desmoplakin I and II** are located in the attachment plaque.

4. **The gap junction (nexus)** occurs at **small discrete sites** for the **metabolic** and **electrical coupling** of cells.
   a. The cell membranes of the two adjoining cells are separated by an intercellular space that is bridged by **connexons.**
      (1) Connexons consist of a transmembrane protein (**connexin**) complex.
      (2) Connexons contain central pores that allow passage of **ions, cyclic adenosine monophosphate (cAMP), amino acids, steroids,** and **small molecules (< 1200 d)** between cells. The opening and closing of the pores is regulated by intracellular levels of calcium.
   b. Gap junctions are also found between **osteocytes, astrocytes, cardiac muscle cells, smooth muscle cells,** and **endocrine cells.**
   c. Cancer cells generally do not have gap junctions, so the cancer cells cannot communicate their mitotic activity to each other, which may explain their uncontrolled growth.

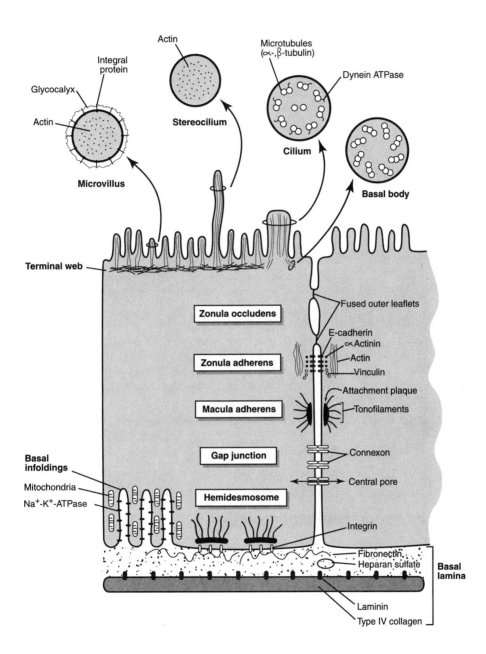

Figure 2-1. Diagram of a hypothetical epithelial cell demonstrating the specializations in the apical, lateral, and basal regions.

C. The basal region

1. **Basal infoldings** are invaginations of the cell membrane that contain **ion pumps** (Na^+-K^+-**ATPase**) found in close association with **mitochondria,** which provide the substrate ATP. Basal infoldings are found in the **proximal and distal convoluted tubules of the kidney** and in **ducts of salivary glands.**

2. **Hemidesmosomes** are junctions that anchor epithelial cells to the underlying basal lamina via a transmembrane protein called **integrin.** As a result, hemidesmosomes provide a connection between the **cytoskeleton** of the epithelial cell and the **extracellular matrix.**

3. Basal lamina

  a. The principal constituents are **fibronectin** (binds to integrin of the hemidesmosome), **heparan sulfate, laminin,** and **type IV collagen.**

  b. **Functions** of the basal lamina include:

   (1) **Forming a barrier** between epithelium and connective tissue

    (a) In **normal conditions,** lymphocytes may pass the basal lamina during immune surveillance.

    (b) In **cancerous conditions,** neoplastic cells may pass the basal lamina during malignant invasion.

   (2) **Serving as a filter** (e.g., renal glomerulus)

   (3) **Playing a role in regeneration** (epithelial, nerve, or muscle cells use the basal lamina as a scaffolding during regeneration or wound healing)

IV. CLINICAL CONSIDERATIONS

A. **Immotile cilia syndrome (Kartagener syndrome)** is a genetic disease involving mutations in genes that code for ciliary proteins (e.g., tubulin, dynein). This results in **situs inversus** (organ reversal due to failure of cells to migrate properly during embryogenesis), **recurrent sinus/pulmonary infections** (inability to move mucous), and **sterility in males** (retarded sperm movement).

B. **Bullous pemphigoid** is an autoimmune disease in which antibodies against **desmosomal proteins** are formed. This results in widespread **skin and mucous membrane blistering** as desmosomes fall apart.

C. **Carcinomas** is a malignant neoplasm derived from epithelium.

D. **Adenocarcinoma** is a malignant neoplasm derived from glandular epithelium.

V. SELECTED PHOTOMICROGRAPHS

A. **Microvilli and cilia** (Figure 2-2; see III A)

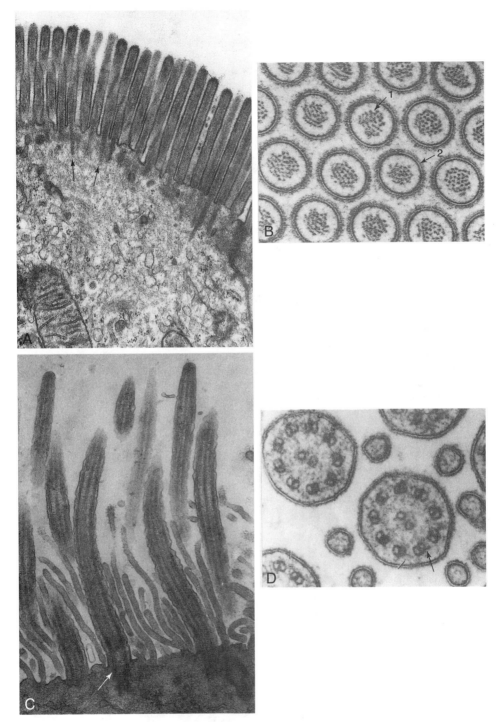

Figure 2-2. (A) Electron micrograph of microvilli comprising the microvillus border of an epithelial cell. Note the actin core (*arrows*) extending into the terminal web within the cytoplasm. (Courtesy of Dr. Jack Brinn, East Carolina University, School of Medicine.) (B) Electron micrograph of microvilli in cross-section demonstrating the actin core (*arrow 1*) and the fuzzy glycocalyx (*arrow 2*). (Courtesy of Dr. A. Ichikawa. Reprinted with permission from Fawcett DW: *A Textbook of Histology*, 12th ed. New York, Chapman Hall, 1994, p 74. Courtesy of Don W. Fawcett, M.D.) (C) Electron micrograph of cilia. Note the microtubule core (*arrow*) extending into the basal body within the cytoplasm. (Courtesy of Dr. Jack Brinn, East Carolina University, School of Medicine.) (D) Electron micrograph of cilia in cross-section. Note the arrangement of microtubules in a 9 + 2 arrangement and the dynein arm (*arrow*). (Reproduced with permission from Simionescu M: *J Cell Biol* 70:608, 1976 by copyright permission of The Rockefeller University Press.)

B. **Zonula occludens** (Figure 2-3; see III B 1)

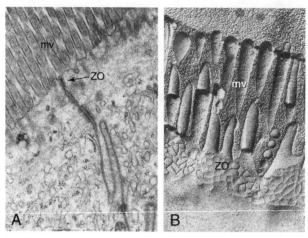

Figure 2-3. (A) In this electron micrograph, fusion between the outer leaflets of two cell membranes can be observed just beneath the microvilli (MV). This type of cell junction is called a zonula occludens (ZO) or tight junction. (Courtesy of Dr. Jack Brinn, East Carolina University, School of Medicine.) (B) A freeze-fracture replica of a zonula occludens or tight junction. A belt-like band of anastomosing strands (ZO) can be observed. The strands are seen as ridges of intramembranous particles on the P-face or complimentary grooves on the E-face. Microvilli (MV) are apparent. (Reprinted with permission from Gilula N: Cell junctions. In *Cell Communication*. Edited by Cox R. New York: John Wiley, 1974, pp 1–29. Reprinted by permission of John Wiley & Sons, Inc.)

C. **Gap junction** (Figure 2-4; see III B 4)

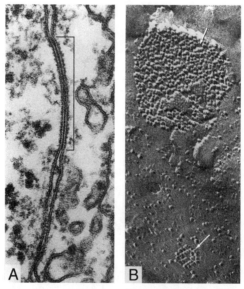

Figure 2-4. (A) In this electron micrograph, the cell junction indicated by the *bracket* is called a gap junction or nexus. (B) A freeze-fracture replica of a gap junction or nexus (*arrows*). Each intramembranous particle located exclusively on the P-face corresponds to a connexon. Gap junctions are constructed from transmembrane proteins (called connexins) that form structures called connexons. Two connexons bridge across the intercellular space to form a channel (or pore) connecting two cells. (Reprinted with permission from Gilula N: Cell junctions. In *Cell Communication*. Edited by Cox R. New York: John Wiley, 1974, pp 1–29. Reprinted by permission of John Wiley & Sons, Inc.)

3

Connective Tissue

I. INTRODUCTION. Types of connective tissue include loose connective tissue (e.g., fascia, lamina propria), dense connective tissue (e.g., tendons), adipose tissue, cartilage, and bone. The common features of all connective tissues are the **ground substance, fibers,** and **cells,** as described below.

II. GROUND SUBSTANCE contains the following components:

    A. Proteoglycans consist of a **core protein,** which binds many side chains of **glycoaminoglycans (GAGs),** and a **link protein,** which binds hyaluronic acid. GAGs are highly sulfated (SO_4^{2-}) and consist of **repeating disaccharide units** of a **hexosamine** (e.g., N-acetylglucosamine, N-acetylgalactosamine) and a **uronic acid** (e.g., glucuronic acid). Specific GAGs include the following.

        1. **Hyaluronic acid** is found in most connective tissues and binds to the link protein of a large number of proteoglycans to form a **proteoglycan aggregate.**

        2. **Chondroitin sulfate** is found in cartilage and bone.

        3. **Keratan sulfate** is found in cartilage and bone, cornea, and intervertebral disk.

        4. **Dermatan sulfate** is found in dermis of skin, blood vessels, and heart valves.

        5. **Heparan sulfate** is found in the basal lamina, lung, and liver.

    B. Glycoproteins

        1. **Fibronectin** is a component of the basal lamina.

        2. **Laminin** is a component of the basal lamina.

        3. **Chondronectin** is found in cartilage.

        4. **Osteocalcin, osteopontin,** and **bone sialoprotein** are found in bone.

    C. The **mineral (inorganic) component** varies depending on the type of connective tissue.

    D. **Water (tissue fluid).** The high concentration of negative charges due to sulfation (SO_4^{2-}) and carboxylation (COO^-) of GAGs attracts water into the ground substance.

III. FIBERS

    A. Collagen contains two characteristic amino acids, **hydroxyproline** and **hydroxylysine.**

        1. **Synthesis of collagen** involves intracellular and extracellular events.

a. Intracellular events include:
  (1) Synthesis of preprocollagen within rough endoplasmic reticulum (rER)
  (2) Hydroxylation of proline and lysine within rER catalyzed by **peptidyl proline hydroxylase** and **peptidyl lysine hydroxylase** (Vitamin C is essential in this step. When vitamin C deficiency [i.e., **scurvy**] occurs, wounds fail to heal, bone formation is impaired, and teeth become loose.)
  (3) Glycosylation of hydroxylysine within rER
  (4) Formation of triple helix **procollagen** within rER (involves registration peptides)
  (5) Addition of carbohydrates within Golgi complex
  (6) Secretion of procollagen
b. Extracellular events include:
  (1) Cleavage of procollagen to form **tropocollagen** by extracellular peptidases
  (2) Self-assembly of tropocollagen into fibrils (**67-nm periodicity**)
  (3) Cross-linking of adjacent tropocollagen molecules catalyzed by **lysyl oxidase**

2. Types of collagen (Table 3-1)

B. **Elastic fibers** consist of an amorphous core of the **elastin** protein surrounded by microfibrils of the **fibrillin** protein. Elastic fibers contain two unique amino acids called **desmosine** and **isodesmosine,** which are involved in cross-linking.

IV. CELLS

A. **Resident or fixed cells** are a stable population of cells that remain in the connective tissue. These include the following types of cells.

1. **Fibroblasts/fibrocytes** are fixed cells that are involved in the secretion of collagen and ground substance.

2. **Macrophages (histiocytes)**
  a. Macrophages arise from **monocytes** within the circulating blood and bone marrow.
  b. They have a **phagocytic function.**

Table 3-1
Distribution of Collagen Types in the Body

Type	Location in Body
I	Fibrocartilage, bone, dermis of skin, tendons In **wound healing,** type I replaces the initial type III collagen. Most ubiquitous type of collagen
II	Hyaline cartilage Elastic cartilage
III	Liver, spleen, tunica media of blood vessels, muscularis externa of gastrointestinal tract In **wound healing,** type III is laid down first. In **keloid formation,** increased amounts of type III are laid down. Traditionally called **reticular fibers**
IV	Basal lamina

(1) **F$_C$ antibody receptors** on the macrophage cell membrane bind antibody-coated foreign material and subsequently phagocytose the material for lysosomal digestion.

(2) **C3 (a component of complement) receptors** on the macrophage cell membrane bind bacteria and subsequently phagocytose the bacteria (called **opsonization**) for lysosomal digestion.

(3) Certain phagocytosed material (e.g., bacilli of tuberculosis and leprosy, *Trypanosoma cruzi*, *Toxoplasma*, *Leishmania*, asbestos) cannot undergo lysosomal digestion, so macrophages will fuse to form **foreign body giant cells.**

(4) In sites of chronic inflammation, macrophages may assemble into epithelial-like sheets called **epithelioid cells of granulomas.**

   c. Macrophages have an **antigen-presenting function.**

(1) **Exogenous antigens** circulating in the bloodstream are phagocytosed by macrophages and undergo degradation in endosomal acid vesicles.

(2) Antigen proteins are degraded into **antigen peptide fragments,** which are presented on the macrophage cell surface in conjunction with class II major histocompatibility complex (MHC).

(3) **CD4+ helper T cells** with antigen-specific T cell receptor (TcR) on its cell surface recognize the antigen peptide fragment.

   d. Macrophages are activated by **lipopolysaccharides** (a surface component of gram-negative bacteria) and **interferon-γ**

   e. They secrete **interleukin-1** (IL-1; stimulates mitosis of T lymphocytes), **interleukin-6** (IL-6; stimulates differentiation of B lymphocytes into plasma cells), **pyrogens** (mediate fever), **tumor necrosis factor-α,** and **granulocyte–macrophage colony-stimulating factor**

3. Mast cells

   a. Mast cells arise from stem cells in the bone marrow.

   b. They have a function in **immediate (type 1) hypersensitivity reactions (anaphylactic reactions).**

   c. They have immunoglobulin E **(IgE) antibody receptors** on their cell membranes that **bind IgE** produced by plasma cells upon **first exposure** to an allergen (e.g., plant pollen, snake venom, foreign serum), which sensitizes the mast cells.

   d. Mast cells secrete the following substances upon **second exposure** to the same allergen, causing the classic wheal-and-flare reaction in the skin:

(1) **Heparin,** an anticoagulant

(2) **Histamine,** which increases vascular permeability and causes smooth muscle contraction of bronchi

(3) **Leukotriene C$_4$ and D$_4$,** which increase vascular permeability, cause vasodilation, and cause smooth muscle contraction of bronchi

(4) **Eosinophil chemotactic factor,** which attracts eosinophils to the inflammation site

4. Adipocytes

   a. Adipocytes in **multilocular (brown) adipose tissue** contain **numerous fat droplets** and **numerous mitochondria that lack elementary particles** on the inner membrane. The energy produced by these mitochondria is dissipated as **heat** instead of being stored as ATP. Brown adipose tissue is present in human **infants after birth** to assist in **regulation of body temperature** but disappears within a few years. Multilocular adipose tissue has a brown color due to the numerous mitochondria that contain **cytochromes,** which have a color similar to hemoglobin.

 b. Adipocytes in **unilocular (white) adipose tissue** contain a **large, single fat droplet** surrounded by a thin rim of cytoplasm. This tissue accounts for all of the stored fat in humans and has a yellow color due to the presence of **carotene.**

  (1) In general, adipocytes synthesize and store **triacylglycerols** (also called triglycerides, fats, or neutral fats), which are composed of **three fatty acids** in ester linkage with **glycerol.**

  (2) **In the fed state,** an increased insulin:glucagon ratio stimulates adipocytes to produce the following reactions.

   (a) Adipocytes **secrete lipoprotein lipase (LPL)** into the capillaries of white adipose tissue. Lipoprotein lipase catalyzes the digestion of triacylglycerols [carried by very low density lipoproteins (VLDL) and chylomicrons] into fatty acids and glycerol. The fatty acids enter the adipocyte to be stored as triacylglycerols. The glycerol travels to the liver.

   (b) Adipocytes **uptake and metabolize glucose** and use it for energy (via glycolysis) and as a source of the glycerol moiety of the stored triacylglycerols.

  (3) **In the fasted state,** a decreased insulin:glucagon ratio and epinephrine stimulate adipocytes to **begin lipolysis** due to increased levels of cyclic adenosine monophosphate (cAMP), which activate **hormone-sensitive lipase.** Hormone-sensitive lipase catalyzes the cleavage of fatty acids from triacylglycerol. The fatty acids become the major fuel of the body because they are used by muscle and kidney for production of energy (i.e., ATP) and converted in the liver to ketone bodies. The glycerol is used as a source of carbon by the liver for gluconeogenesis.

  (4) Adipocytes secrete a hormone called **leptin** that has an **anorexic action** in that leptin **decreases appetite** and **decreases body weight** (due exclusively to a reduction of fat stores). The action of leptin is mediated through satiety centers in the **hypothalamus** (i.e., **paraventricular and arcuate nuclei**) where **leptin receptors** are found. The gene for leptin has been cloned and is called the **LEP gene** in humans.

 5. **Chondroblasts and chondrocytes** are discussed in Chapter 4.

 6. **Osteoblasts and osteocytes** are discussed in Chapter 5.

B. **Transient or free cells** enter connective tissue from blood, usually during inflammation. These cells include **neutrophils, eosinophils, basophils, monocytes, B lymphocytes, plasma cells,** and **T lymphocytes,** which are discussed in Chapter 9.

V. CLINICAL CONSIDERATIONS

 A. **Ehlers-Danlos syndrome** is a genetic defect involving **peptidyl lysine hydroxylase** that affects **type I and type III collagen** synthesis, resulting in hypermobile joints, excessive stretchability of the skin, and rupture of large bowel and/or large arteries.

 B. **Marfan syndrome** is a genetic defect involving **fibrillin** (a component of **elastic fibers**), resulting in weakened tunica media of aorta (aortic dissection) and ectopia lentis.

 C. **Homocystinuria** is a genetic defect involving the enzyme **cystathionine synthetase,** resulting in abnormal cross-linking of collagen.

 D. **Osteogenesis imperfecta** is a genetic defect involving **type I collagen,** resulting in spontaneous fractures of bone and blue sclera of the eye.

 E. **Alport syndrome (hereditary nephritis)** is a genetic defect involving **type IV collagen,** resulting in renal failure and deafness.

F. **Keloid formation** is a deviation in normal wound healing whereby an excessive accumulation of collagen occurs, resulting in a raised, tumorous scar.

G. **Amyloidosis** is a group of diseases that have in common the **deposition of amyloid** (a proteinaceous substance) in the intercellular space of various organs.

1. By light microscopy, amyloid is an eosinophilic, amorphous substance. By electron microscopy, amyloid is composed of **nonbranching fibrillar proteins** (95%) and a glycoprotein called **P component,** which is pentagonal in shape (5%).

2. A number of different nonbranching fibrillar proteins have been identified, which include:

a. **Amyloid light chain,** an immunoglobulin protein secreted by plasma cells

b. **Amyloid-associated** protein, synthesized by the liver

c. **Beta$_2$-microglobulin,** a component of the major histocompatibility complex class I proteins

d. **Beta$_2$-amyloid,** a 4000-d peptide

e. **Islet amyloid polypeptide (amylin),** which is increased within pancreatic islets of Langerhans in patients with type 2 diabetes

3. **Types of amyloidosis** include the following.

a. **Immunocyte dyscrasias with amyloidosis (primary amyloidosis)** is the most common form of amyloidosis and is associated with the **amyloid light chain protein.** Some patients with **multiple myeloma** (a plasma cell neoplasia) demonstrate amyloidosis along with the presence of light chains (**Bence Jones proteins**) in the serum and urine.

b. **Reactive systemic amyloidosis (secondary amyloidosis)** occurs as a secondary complication to **chronic inflammation** (e.g., rheumatoid arthritis, regional enteritis, ulcerative colitis) and is associated with the **amyloid-associated protein.**

c. **Hemodialysis-associated amyloidosis** occurs in patients on **long-term hemodialysis** and is associated with the **beta$_2$-microglobulin protein.**

d. **Senile cerebral amyloidosis** occurs in patients with **Alzheimer disease** and is associated with **beta$_2$-amyloid protein** deposition in cerebral plaques.

e. **Endocrine amyloid** occurs in patients with **type 2 diabetes** and is associated with **islet amyloid polypeptide** deposition in the pancreatic islets.

VI. SELECTED PHOTOMICROGRAPHS

A. Proteoglycan aggregate (Figure 3-1; see II A)

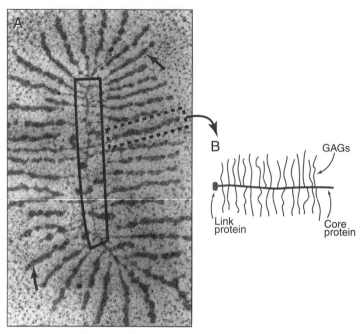

Figure 3-1.   (A) Electron micrograph of a proteoglycan aggregate. A proteoglycan aggregate consists of a large number of proteoglycans (*dotted box* indicates one proteoglycan) bound to hyaluronic acid (*boxed area*). The thick, fuzzy areas (*arrows*) indicate the side chains of glycosaminoglycans (GAGs). (Reproduced with permission from Buckwalter JA, Rosenberg L: Structural changes during development in bovine fetal epiphyseal cartilage. *Collagen Relat Res* 3:489, 1983.) (B) A diagram of a proteoglycan showing the core protein, which binds many side chains of GAGs, and a link protein, which binds hyaluronic acid.

B. Collagen and elastic fibers (Figure 3-2; see III A–B)

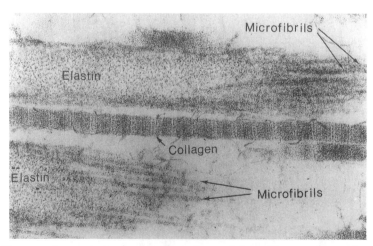

Figure 3-2.   Electron micrograph showing a collagen fiber and elastic fibers consisting of an amorphous core of elastin protein and microfibrils of the fibrillin protein. Note the 67-nm periodicity of collagen. (Reprinted with permission from Fawcett DW: *A Textbook of Histology*, 12th ed. New York, Chapman Hall, 1994, p 147. Courtesy of J. C. Fanning.)

4

Cartilage

I. INTRODUCTION. Cartilage is a type of connective tissue that includes **hyaline cartilage** (e.g., articular ends of long bones), **elastic cartilage** (e.g., pinna of ear), and **fibrocartilage** (e.g., annulus fibrosus of the intervertebral disk). Cartilage has all the common features of connective tissue, which include ground substance, fibers, and cells as indicated below.

II. GROUND SUBSTANCE consists of:

A. **Proteoglycans,** containing side chains of glycosaminoglycans (GAGs), specifically **chondroitin sulfate** and **keratan sulfate**

B. **Glycoproteins,** including **chondronectin** and **chondrocalcin** (a calcium-binding protein)

C. **No mineral (inorganic) component,** because cartilage is not mineralized

D. **Water (tissue fluid)**—high degree of hydration (75%)

III. FIBERS

A. **Type I collagen** is found in fibrocartilage.

B. **Type II collagen** is found in hyaline and elastic cartilage.

IV. CELLS

A. **Chondrogenic cells** are found in the perichondrium, where they undergo mitosis and differentiate into chondroblasts.

B. **Chondroblasts** arise from chondrogenic cells and may undergo mitosis.

C. **Chondrocytes** reside in **lacunae.** They form **isogenous groups** that are surrounded by a **territorial matrix** that stains basophilic due to the higher local concentration of chondroitin sulfate. Chondrocytes may undergo mitosis.

V. BLOOD VESSELS AND NERVES are absent. Like epithelium, cartilage is avascular. It receives its nutrients by diffusion through the ground substance.

VI. CHONDROGENESIS occurs in the embryo when mesodermal cells withdraw their processes and condense into aggregations called **centers of chondrification.** Cartilage may then grow in the following ways:

A. **Interstitial growth** occurs by mitosis of preexisting chondrocytes.

B. **Appositional growth** occurs by differentiation of chondrogenic cells in the perichondrium into chondroblasts.

VII. HORMONAL INFLUENCE

A. **Triiodothyronine (T_3), thyroxine (T_4), testosterone, and growth hormone** (via somatomedin C) stimulate cartilage growth.

B. **Cortisone, hydrocortisone, and estradiol** inhibit cartilage growth.

VIII. REPAIR.
In the adult, damaged cartilage shows limited repair (regeneration) and may form scar tissue instead of cartilage. In young children, damaged cartilage shows a greater capacity for repair.

5
Bone

I. INTRODUCTION. Bone is a type of connective tissue that has a **supportive and protective function** and also serves as a **reservoir for calcium and phosphate.** Bone has all the common features of connective tissue, which include ground substance, fibers, and cells, as indicated below.

II. GROUND SUBSTANCE consists of:

   A. Proteoglycans containing a side chain of glycosaminoglycans (GAGs), specifically **chondroitin sulfate** and **keratan sulfate**

   B. Glycoproteins, such as **osteonectin, osteocalcin** (a calcium-binding protein), and **osteopontin**

   C. A mineral (inorganic) component that includes **hydroxyapatite** (calcium phosphate crystals), **citrate ions,** and **bicarbonate ions**

   1. The mineral component comprises approximately 75% of the bone mass and contributes to the **hardness/rigidity** of bone.

   2. A dilute acid or chelating agent, such as ethylenediaminetetraacetic acid (EDTA) demineralizes bone.

   D. Water (tissue fluid), which contributes to a low degree of hydration (7%)

III. FIBERS consist of **type I collagen** that provides **tensile strength** to bone.

IV. CELLS

   A. Osteoprogenitor cells differentiate into osteoblasts during osteogenesis and bone repair and may undergo mitosis.

   B. Osteoblasts

   1. Osteoblasts are derived from osteoprogenitor cells.

   2. They secrete **osteoid,** which is unmineralized bone matrix consisting of proteoglycans, glycoproteins, and type I collagen.
      a. For mineralization to occur, osteoblasts secrete **osteocalcin** and **alkaline phosphatase,** which hydrolyzes phosphate-containing substrates as well as calcium β-glycerophosphate to release calcium and phosphate.
      b. In addition, osteoblasts release **matrix vesicles** (membrane-bound vesicles), which concentrate calcium and phosphate and are the most important factor necessary for mineralization to occur.

    c. The **blood alkaline phosphatase level** can be monitored clinically to assess osteogenesis or bone repair.

  3. Osteoblasts secrete **interleukin-1 (IL-1),** which is a potent stimulator of osteoclast activity.

  4. They have **parathyroid hormone receptors** and **1,25-dihydroxyvitamin D$_3$** [i.e., 1,25-(OH)$_2$ vitamin D] **receptors.**

  5. Osteoblasts do not undergo mitosis.

C. Osteocytes

  1. Osteocytes and their cytoplasmic processes are surrounded by bone matrix because they reside in spaces called **lacunae** and **canaliculi,** respectively. Cytoplasmic processes of neighboring osteocytes communicate via **gap junctions.**

  2. Osteocytes do not undergo mitosis.

D. Osteoclasts

  1. Osteoclasts are derived from **granulocyte-monocyte progenitor cells** within the bone marrow.

  2. They are multinucleated cells that reside in shallow depressions of the bone called **Howship's lacunae.**

  3. They function in **bone resorption** in the following ways:
    a. Secrete **lysosomal enzymes** (e.g., β-glucuronidase, aryl sulfatase) to digest the proteoglycans of the bone matrix
    b. Secrete **collagenase** to digest type I collagen of the bone matrix
      (1) The **urine hydroxyproline level** can be monitored clinically to assess bone resorption.
      (2) Hydroxyproline is an amino acid that is unique to collagen.

  4. Osteoclasts have a **ruffled border** (infoldings of the cell membrane) closest to the bone that contains Na$^+$-K$^+$-ATPase and **carbonic anhydrase,** which produces hydrogen ions that create an acid environment to digest the mineral component of the bone matrix.

  5. They have **calcitonin receptors.**

  6. They do not undergo mitosis.

V. BLOOD VESSELS AND NERVES are present in **Haversian canals** and **Volkmann's canals.** However, they are absent in lacunae and canaliculi.

VI. OSTEOGENESIS always occurs by replacing preexisting connective tissue. In the embryo, two types of osteogenesis occur:

A. **Intramembranous ossification** occurs in the embryo when mesoderm condenses into sheets of highly vascular **connective tissue,** which then forms a primary ossification center. Bones that form via intramembranous ossification include **flat bones of the skull.**

B. **Endochondral ossification** occurs in the embryo when mesoderm initially forms a **hyaline cartilage** model, which then develops a primary ossification center at the diaphysis. Later, secondary ossification centers form at the epiphysis at each end of the bone. Bones that form via endochondral ossification include the **humerus, femur, tibia,** and **other long bones.**

1. **Growth in length of long bones** occurs at the **epiphyseal plate,** which includes a number of zones as indicated below.

   a. The **zone of reserve** contains resting chondrocytes.

   b. The **zone of proliferation** contains chondrocytes undergoing mitosis and forming isogenous groups.

   c. The **zone of hypertrophy** contains hypertrophied chondrocytes, which secrete alkaline phosphatase to increase calcium and phosphate levels.

   d. The **zone of calcification** contains dead chondrocytes and calcified cartilage matrix called **spicules.**

   e. The **zone of ossification** contains osteoprogenitor cells that congregate on spicules and differentiate into osteoblasts. Osteoblasts deposit bone on the surface of a spicule to form a **mixed spicule,** which consists of calcified cartilage matrix and bone.

2. **Growth in diameter of long bones** occurs at the **diaphysis** by deposition of bone at the periphery (**appositional growth**) as osteoprogenitor cells within the **periosteum** differentiate into osteoblasts.

VII. BONE REPAIR.
In the adult, bone shows a **high capacity** for repair through the proliferation of osteoprogenitor cells. After a bone fracture, the following actions take place.

A. Ruptured blood vessels form a **hematoma,** which bridges the fracture gap and provides a meshwork for the influx of inflammatory cells that secrete products (e.g., transforming growth factor β; fibroblast growth factor) to activate osteoprogenitor cells to form osteoblasts.

B. After 1 week, the hematoma is organized into a **soft tissue callus (procallus)** that anchors the ends of the fracture but provides no rigidity for weight bearing.

C. Osteoblasts begin to deposit **immature woven bone.** Woven bone is formed whenever osteoblasts produce osteoid rapidly and is characterized by an irregular arrangement of collagen.

D. Mesenchymal cells in the procallus form **hyaline cartilage** at the periphery that envelops the fracture site. The hyaline cartilage undergoes endochondral ossification.

E. The collection of bone at the fracture is now called a **bony callus.** As the bony callus mineralizes, controlled weight bearing can be tolerated.

F. Eventually all the woven bone of the bony callus is remodeled into **mature lamellar bone.** Lamellar bone is characterized by a regular layered arrangement of collagen.

VIII. HORMONAL INFLUENCE

A. **Parathyroid hormone** (a protein hormone) acts directly on osteoblasts to secrete **IL-1,** which stimulates osteoclasts to **increase bone resorption,** thereby **elevating blood calcium levels.**

B. **1,25-(OH)$_2$ vitamin D** (a steroid hormone) acts directly on osteoblasts to secrete **IL-1,** which stimulates osteoclasts to **increase bone resorption,** thereby **elevating blood calcium levels.**

C. **Calcitonin** acts directly on osteoclasts to **decrease bone resorption,** thereby **lowering blood calcium levels.**

D. **Growth hormone** promotes skeletal growth and bone remodeling.

E. **Estrogens and androgens.** The closure of the epiphyseal plate is closely related to the development of the ovaries and testes.

1. In patients with **precocious sexual development,** skeletal growth is stunted due to premature closure of the epiphyseal plate.

2. In patients with **gonadal hypoplasia,** closure of the epiphyseal plate is delayed, and arms or legs become disproportionately long.

F. **Thyroid hormones.** Triiodothyronine and thyroxine stimulate endochondral ossification and linear growth of bone.

G. **Cortisol** inhibits bone formation.

IX. CLINICAL CONSIDERATIONS

A. **Primary osteoporosis (senile or postmenopausal)** is a critical **loss of bone mass** associated with a deficiency of either **growth hormone** (senile) or **estrogen** (postmenopausal). Decreased estrogen levels result in increased secretion of IL-1 (a potent stimulator of osteoclasts) from monocytes. Osteoporosis is widely recognized as a serious consequence of chronic glucocorticoid use to manage diseases including rheumatoid arthritis, inflammatory bowel diseases (e.g., Crohn's disease), asthma, emphysema, and rejection of organ transplant. Although all glucocorticoid users are at risk of bone loss, postmenopausal women are at a particularly high risk for glucocorticoid-induced osteoporosis and its fractures.

B. **Acromegaly** is characterized by thick bones as a result of **excess growth hormone.**

C. **Paget's disease**

1. Paget's disease is characterized by **uncontrolled osteoclast activity,** causing widespread bone resorption followed by intense osteoblast activity, producing woven bone that fills in the erosion.

2. The net effect is paradoxically an increase in bone mass that is architecturally unsound because the woven bone persists.

D. **Osteomalacia** (in adults) **and rickets** (in children)

1. Osteomalacia and rickets are characterized by **lack of minerals within osteoid,** which occurs as a result of **vitamin D deficiency.**

2. To understand osteomalacia and rickets, **normal vitamin D metabolism** must be explained as indicated below:

   a. Vitamin D sources include dietary intake and production by skin keratinocytes stimulated by ultraviolet light.

   b. Vitamin D is hydroxylated by liver hepatocytes to 25-hydroxyvitamin D [i.e., 25-(OH) vitamin D].

   c. 25-(OH) vitamin D is hydroxylated in the kidney to **1,25-$(OH)_2$ vitamin D,** the active metabolite that functions similar to a steroid hormone.

   d. 1,25-$(OH)_2$D **stimulates absorption of calcium and phosphate ions** from the intestinal lumen into the blood, thereby **elevating blood calcium and phosphate levels.** Calcium and phosphate are used in the normal mineralization of osteoid.

3. Physical signs of osteomalacia in adults include **bowed legs, increased tendency to fracture,** and **scoliotic deformity of the vertebral column.**

4. Physical signs of rickets in nonambulatory children include **craniotabes** (elastic recoil of the skull upon compression), **"rachitic rosary"** (excess osteoid at the costochondral junction), and **"pigeon-breast deformity"** (anterior protrusion of sternum).

E. Scurvy

1. Scurvy is characterized by **lack of collagen within osteoid,** which occurs as a result of **vitamin C deficiency.**

2. **Vitamin C** is necessary for the hydroxylation of proline and lysine amino acids during collagen synthesis.

3. Physical signs of scurvy include **poor bone growth** and **poor fracture repair** due to lack of collagen within osteoid, as well as **hemorrhages** in the skin (purpura), gingival mucosa, and joints due to a weakened tunica media of blood vessels.

F. **Vitamin A.** An excess of vitamin A causes a premature closure of the epiphyseal plate, resulting in a person of small stature.

X. CARTILAGE AND BONE COMPARISON (Table 5-1)

Table 5-1
Cartilage and Bone Comparison

Characteristic	Cartilage	Bone
Ground substance	Chondroitin sulfate, keratan sulfate Chondronectin, chondrocalcin No mineralization High degree of hydration (75%)	Chondroitin sulfate, keratan sulfate Osteonectin, osteocalcin, osteoporin Hydroxyapatite, citrate, bicarbonate Low degree of hydration (7%)
Fibers	Type I collagen (fibrocartilage) Type II collagen (hyaline and elastic)	Type I collagen (provides tensile strength)
Vascularity	Avascular; nutrients received via diffusion	Highly vascular
Nerves	Absent	Present
Growth	Interstitial and appositional	Appositional only
Repair	Low	High
Mitosis	Chondrogenic—yes Chondroblasts—yes Chondrocytes—yes	Osteoprogenitor—yes Osteoblasts—no Osteocytes—no Osteoclasts—no
Communication	No junctions between chondrocytes	Gap junctions between osteocytes
Hormonal influence	T_3, T_4, testosterone, GH, cortisone, hydrocortisone, estradiol	PTH; 1,25-$(OH)_2$ vitamin D; calcitonin; GH; estrogens; androgens; T_3; T_4; cortisol
Vitamin influence	N/A	Vitamins D, C, and A

T_3 = triiodothyronine; T_4 = thyroxine; GH = growth hormone; PTH = parathyroid hormone; 1,25-$(OH)_2$ vitamin D = 1,25-dihydroxyvitamin D_3.

XI. SELECTED PHOTOMICROGRAPHS

A. Spongy bone and compact bone (Figure 5-1)

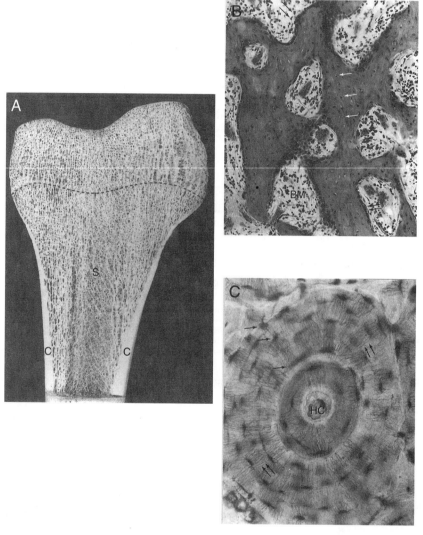

Figure 5-1.   (A) Coronal section through the epiphysis of an adult tibia. Gross anatomically, two different types of bone can be described: spongy bone (S) arranged as trabeculae that are adapted to mechanical forces, and compact bone (C) forming a rigid outer shell. The *dotted line* is the site of the former epiphyseal plate. (Reprinted with permission from Rohen JW, Yokochi C, Lutjen-Drecoll E: *Color Atlas of Anatomy,* 4th ed. Baltimore, Williams and Wilkins, 1998, p 9.) (B) Light micrograph of spongy bone [hematoxylin–eosin (HE) stained section]. Trabeculae of spongy bone are shown with a lamellar (layered linearly) arrangement of osteocytes (*single arrows*) and bone matrix. Osteoblasts (*double arrows*) can be observed on the surface of the trabeculae. The interstices between the trabeculae are filled with bone marrow (BM). (C) Light micrograph of compact bone (ground bone section). An osteon or Haversian system of compact bone is shown with a lamellar (layered concentrically) arrangement of osteocytes within lacunae (*single arrows*) and bone matrix. Osteocytes have many cytoplasmic processes within canaliculi (*double arrows*) that extend throughout the bone matrix and communicate with other osteocytes. Within the center of an osteon is a Haversian canal (HC) that contains blood vessels and nerves.

B. Osteoclast (Figure 5-2; see IV D)

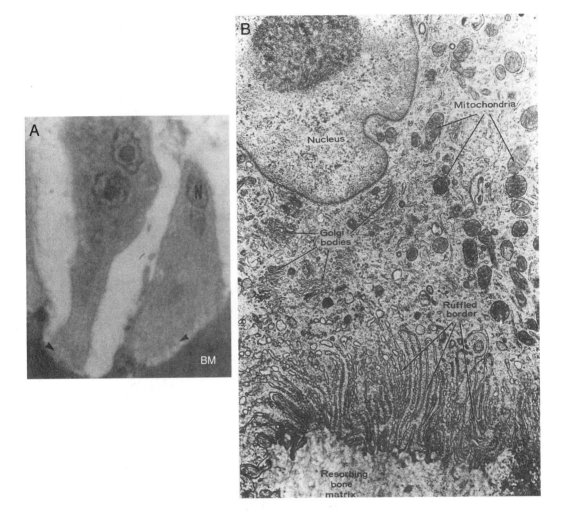

Figure 5-2. (A) Light micrograph of osteoclasts. Two osteoclasts are shown attached to bone matrix (BM). The ruffled border is shown (*arrowheads*). N = Nucleus. (Reprinted with permission from Holliger J: Cartilage and bone. In: *Color Atlas of Histology*, 2nd ed. Edited by Gartner LP, Hiatt JL. Baltimore, Williams and Wilkins, 1994, p 78.) (B) Electron micrograph of an osteoclast. The cell membrane contains calcitonin receptors and a ruffled border adjacent to the resorbing bone matrix. (Reprinted with permission from Garrant P: Bone. In: A *Textbook of Histology*, 12th ed. Edited by Fawcett DW. New York, Chapman Hall, 1994, p 210. Courtesy of P. Garrant.)

C. Epiphyseal growth plate (Figure 5-3; see VIII E)

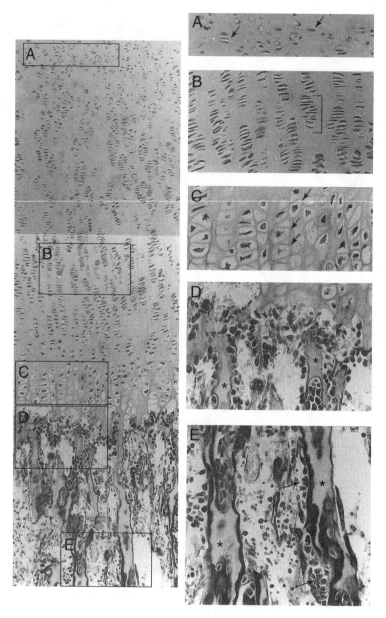

Figure 5-3. Light micrograph of endochondral ossification at the epiphyseal plate. (A) Zone of reserve consists of hyaline cartilage and chondrocytes (*arrows*). (B) Zone of proliferation consists of hyaline cartilage and chondrocytes undergoing mitosis forming stacks of chondrocytes (*bracket*). (C) Zone of hypertrophy consists of hyaline cartilage and hypertrophied chondrocytes (*arrows*) that are secreting alkaline phosphatase to increase calcium and phosphate levels in the ground substance. (D) Zone of calcification consists of dead chondrocytes and calcified cartilage matrix called spicules (*asterisk*). (E) Zone of ossification consists of osteoprogenitor cells in the marrow cavity that differentiate into osteoblasts (*arrows*). Osteoblasts deposit bone (*black areas*) on the surface of a spicule to form a mixed spicule (*asterisk*).

6

Muscle

I. SKELETAL MUSCLE. The terms muscle fiber and muscle cell are synonymous.

    A. Fiber (cell) types. Skeletal muscle fibers can be classified mainly into **red (type I)** and **white (type II)** fibers that have quite different characteristics based on their function (Table 6-1).

        1. **Red fibers** are **slow-twitch** fibers and are largely present, for example, in the long muscles of the back (antigravity muscles).

        2. **White fibers** are **fast-twitch** fibers and are largely present, for example, in the extraocular muscles of the eye.

    B. **Cross-striations** (Figure 6-1)

        1. The **A band** contains both thin and thick myofilaments and is the **dark band** seen when using an electron microscope.

        2. The **I band** contains only thin myofilaments and is the **light band** seen when using an electron microscope.

        3. The **H band** bisects the A band and contains only thick myofilaments.

Table 6-1
Characteristics of Muscle Fiber

Characteristic	Red Fiber	White Fiber
Speed of contraction	Slow	Fast
Myoglobin content*	High	Low
Generation of ATP	Aerobic glycolysis[†] Oxidative phosphorylation	Anaerobic glycolysis[†]
Number of mitochondria	Many	Few
Glycogen content	Low	High
Succinate dehydrogenase NADH dehydrogenase	High	Low
Glycolytic enzymes	Low	High

*Myoglobin is an oxygen-binding protein similar to hemoglobin and accounts for the reddish appearance of red (type I) fibers.
[†]Aerobic glycolysis (conversion of glucose to carbon dioxide and water) is a relatively slow process so that it can meet the demands of red fibers, but it yields 36 to 38 moles of ATP per mole of glucose.
[†]Anaerobic glycolysis (conversion of glucose to lactate) is a relatively fast process so that it can meet the demands of white fibers, but it yields only 2 moles of ATP per mole of glucose.
NADH = reduced nicotinamide adenine dinucleotide.

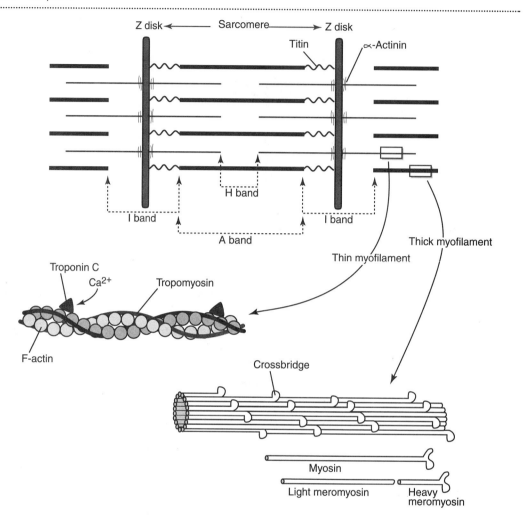

Figure 6-1. Organization of thin and thick myofilaments in skeletal muscle.

4. The **Z disk** bisects the I band. The distance between two Z disks delimits a **sarcomere,** which is the basic unit of contraction for the myofibril. The Z disk contains **α-actinin,** which anchors thin filaments to the Z disk.

C. Thin myofilaments

1. **F actin** has an active site that interacts with the **cross-bridges** of myosin.

2. **Tropomyosin** blocks the active site on F actin during relaxation.

3. **Troponin C** is a calcium-binding protein.

D. Thick myofilaments

1. **Myosin** can be cleaved by trypsin into **light meromyosin** and **heavy meromyosin,**

which contains **crossbridges.** The cross-bridges have **actin-binding sites** and **ATPase** activity.

2. **Titin** anchors myosin to the Z disks and helps the muscle to accommodate extreme stretching.

E. **Changes in contracted and stretched muscle.** The cross-striational pattern of skeletal muscle changes when it is contracted or stretched. These changes are caused by the degree of interdigitation of the thin and thick myofilaments (Table 6-2).

F. **Contraction of skeletal muscle** (Figure 6-2)

1. A triad consists of a **transverse tubule (T tubule)** located at the **A-I junction** flanked on either side by two **terminal cisternae.**
   a. A T tubule is an invagination of the cell membrane and transmits an action potential to the depths of a muscle cell.
   b. Terminal cisternae are dilated sacs of sarcoplasmic reticulum that store, release, and reaccumulate calcium ions.

2. In response to an action potential, calcium ions are released from the terminal cisternae.

3. Calcium ions bind to troponin, which allows the **myosin crossbridge–ADP–phosphate complex** to bind to actin. Repetitive action potentials may produce saturating levels of calcium ions for troponin and thereby cause **tetany.**

4. ADP–phosphate is released, leaving the myosin crossbridge bound to actin.

5. The myosin crossbridge binds ATP, which detaches the myosin crossbridge from actin. (If ATP is not available, the muscle will not relax, and **rigor mortis** results.)

6. ATP is hydrolyzed by myosin ATPase, and the products (ADP and phosphate) remain bound to the myosin crossbridge, thereby reforming the myosin crossbridge–ADP–phosphate complex.

G. **Neuromuscular junction** (also called **myoneural junction** or **motor endplate**)

1. Synaptic terminals of alpha motoneurons contain synaptic vesicles, which store **acetylcholine (ACh).** ACh is synthesized by the condensation of **acetyl CoA** and

Table 6-2
Changes in Contracted and Stretched Muscle

Band	Change Compared with Relaxed Muscle	
	Contracted	Stretched
A band	No change	No change
I band	Shortens	Lenghtens
H band	Shortens	Lengthens
Z disks	Move closer together	Move farther apart
Receptors		
Muscle spindle	Shortens	Lengthens
Golgi tendon organ	Moves closer together	Moves farther apart

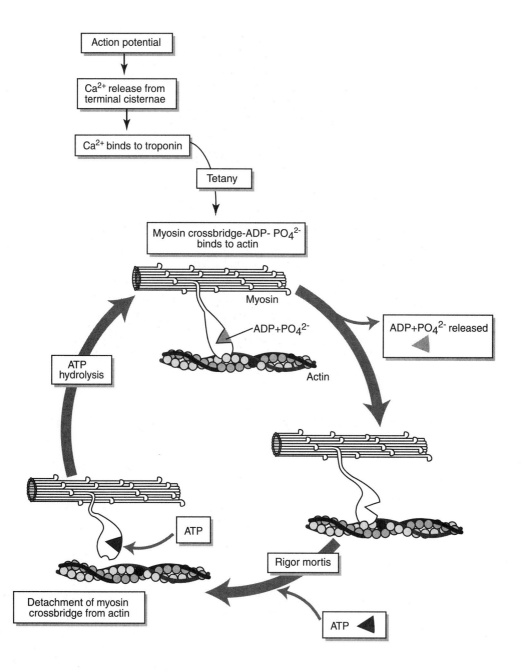

Figure 6-2. Events in skeletal muscle contraction. Note the points where tetany and rigor mortis occur.

choline, which is catalyzed by **choline-O-acetyltransferase.** Choline is obtained by active uptake from the extracellular fluid.

2. The cell membrane of the synaptic terminal is called the **presynaptic membrane** and is where exocytotic release of ACh occurs. The cell membrane of the muscle fiber is called the **postsynaptic membrane,** and it contains the **nicotinic acetylcholine receptor (nAChR).**

3. The space between the presynaptic and postsynaptic membrane is called the **synaptic cleft,** and it contains the basal lamina associated with the enzyme **acetylcholinesterase (AChE),** which hydrolyzes ACh into acetate and choline.

4. nAChR is a **transmitter-gated ion channel** such that when nAChR binds ACh, the "gate" is opened and allows an **influx of sodium ions.** This influx causes depolarization of the postsynaptic membrane called the **endplate potential.**

5. Endplate potentials spread to areas of the muscle fiber cell membrane and T tubule by **electrotonic conduction** until a threshold is reached and an action potential is generated. (Note: An action potential is not generated at the neuromuscular junction itself.)

6. **α-Bungarotoxin** (a snake venom **α-toxin**) and **curare** (a plant toxin) bind to nAChR, thereby preventing ACh from binding.

H. Innervation. A single axon of an **alpha motoneuron** may innervate 1 to 5 muscle fibers (forming a small motor unit), or the axon may branch and innervate >150 muscle fibers (forming a large motor unit). A **motor unit** (not a muscle fiber) is the functional contractile unit of a muscle.

I. Denervation. If a nerve to a muscle is severed, muscle **fasciculations** (small irregular contractions) occur caused by release of ACh from the degenerating axon. Several days after denervation, muscle **fibrillations** (spontaneous repetitive contractions) occur caused by a supersensitivity of the muscle to ACh as ACh receptors spread out over the entire cell membrane of the muscle fiber.

J. Skeletal muscle repair (regeneration) is limited. Skeletal muscle fibers develop embryologically from **rhabdomyoblasts.** After injury or extensive exercise, **satellite cells** present in the adult proliferate and fuse to form new skeletal muscle fibers. Adult skeletal muscle fibers do not undergo mitosis.

K. Stretch (sensory) receptors

1. **Muscle spindles** activate the **myotatic (stretch) reflex** and consist of **nuclear bag fibers** or **nuclear chain fibers.**
  a. **Nuclear bag fibers** contain nuclei that are bunched together centrally and that transmit sensory information to **group Ia afferent neurons.**
  b. **Nuclear chain fibers** contain nuclei that are linearly arranged and that transmit sensory information (muscle length and rate of change in muscle length) to **group Ia** and **group II** afferent neurons.
  c. Nuclear bag fibers and nuclear chain fibers are innervated by **γ-motoneurons** that set the sensitivity of the muscle spindle. The activity of γ-motoneurons is controlled by descending pathways of higher brain centers (upper motoneurons) such that after spinal cord transection, hyperactivity of γ-motoneurons plays a role in muscle **spasticity** and muscle **hypertonia.**

2. **Golgi tendon organs** activate the **inverse myotatic (stretch) reflex** and consist of a bundle of collagen fibers within the muscle **tendon** that transmit sensory information (force on the muscle) to **group Ib afferent neurons.**

L. Clinical considerations

 1. **Duchenne muscular dystrophy (DMD)** is a genetic disease that shows **X-linked recessive inheritance.**

 a. The DMD gene is located on the short (p) arm of chromosome X in band 21 (i.e., **Xp21**) and encodes for the **dystrophin** protein.

 b. Dystrophin anchors within skeletal muscle fibers to the extracellular matrix, thereby stabilizing the cell membrane.

 c. A mutation of the DMD gene alters the normal function of dystrophin, leading to **progressive muscle weakness and wasting.**

 2. **Myasthenia gravis** is an **autoimmune disease** characterized by circulating antibodies against the ACh receptor (anti-AChR) and decreased number of ACh receptors.

 a. It is characterized by muscle weakness that fluctuates daily or even within hours.

 b. The extraocular muscles are generally involved, with **ptosis** and **diplopia** being the first disability.

II. CARDIAC MUSCLE

A. Cardiac myocytes

 1. Cardiac myocytes contract through intrinsic action potentials that are passed to neighboring cells by gap junctions; that is, the heart beat is **myogenic.**

 2. Cardiac myocytes contain a **diad,** which consists of a **T tubule** located at the Z disk and flanked by one **terminal cisterna.**

 3. The ends of neighboring cardiac myocytes have interdigitating cell surfaces that are attached by **intercalated disks,** which consist of a **fascia adherens, desmosomes,** and **gap junctions.**

B. **Purkinje myocytes** are **modified cardiac myocytes** that are specialized for conduction and are joined with neighboring Purkinje myocytes by extensive gap junctions. Purkinje myocytes are not neurons.

C. **Cardiac muscle repair (regeneration)** is virtually nonexistent. Injured cardiac myocytes (e.g., myocardial infarction) are generally replaced by connective tissue.

III. SMOOTH MUSCLE

A. **Smooth muscle fibers (cells)** have the following characteristics:

 1. They have **cytoplasmic dense bodies** (equivalent to **Z disks**), which contain **α-actinin**

 2. Smooth muscle fibers have **subplasmalemmal dense plaques,** which contain **vinculin** and **talin**

 3. Smooth muscle fibers contain **actin** and **myosin** filaments, as well as **desmin** and **vimentin** intermediate filaments (Vimentin is found predominately in vascular smooth muscle.)

 4. They have numerous invaginations of the cell membrane called **caveolae** (equivalent to **T tubules**)

5. They use the protein **calmodulin** to bind calcium

6. Smooth muscle fibers synthesize many extracellular components such as laminin, collagen, and elastin

B. **Contraction mechanisms**

1. **Intrinsic.** Smooth muscle fibers of the **gastrointestinal tract** contract through **intrinsically generated** excitations that are passed to neighboring cells by **gap junctions.** Postganglionic autonomic neurons only modify the intrinsic activity.

2. **Neural.** Smooth muscle fibers of the **large arteries, ciliary muscle and iris of the eye, and ductus deferens** contract through neural excitations generated by postganglionic autonomic neurons that pass over the muscle surface and synapse en passant. No neuromuscular junctions are present as in skeletal muscle.

3. **Hormonal. Myoepithelial cells of the mammary gland** and **smooth muscle fibers of the myometrium** contract through hormonal excitations generated by **oxytocin** secreted from the **neurohypophysis. Epinephrine** and **norepinephrine** also stimulate smooth muscle fiber contraction.

C. **Smooth muscle repair (regeneration)** is very high.

IV. COMPARISONS AND CONTRASTS (Table 6-3)

Table 6-3
Comparison of Muscle Types

Characteristic	Muscle Type		
	Skeletal	**Cardiac**	**Smooth**
Nucleus	Multinucleated; peripheral location	Single nucleus; central location	Single nucleus; central location
Bands	A and I bands	A and I bands	Absent
Z disks	Present	Present	Absent; dense bodies are present
T tubules	Present	Present	Absent; caveolae are present
Cell junctions	Absent	Absent	Gap junctions
Neuromuscular junction	Present	Absent; contraction is intrinsic	Absent; contraction is intrinsic, neural, or hormonal
Stretch receptors	Present	Absent	Absent
Calcium ion binding	Troponin	Troponin	Calmodulin
Regeneration	Limited	None	High

V. SELECTED PHOTOMICROGRAPHS

A. Skeletal muscle (Figure 6-3; see I B)

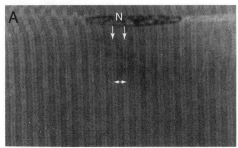

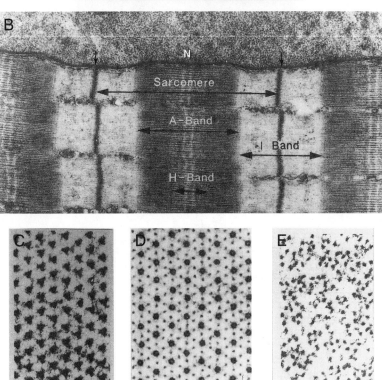

Figure 6-3. (A) Light micrograph of skeletal muscle cut longitudinally. Note the A band (*dark*) and I band (*light*). The I band is bisected by the Z disk (*arrows*). A sarcomere (Z disk to Z disk) is indicated by the *double-headed arrow*. A peripherally located nucleus (N) is shown. (B) Electron micrograph of skeletal muscle cut longitudinally. Note the A band (dark) and I band (*light*) and H band. The I band is bisected by the Z disk (*single-headed arrows*). A sarcomere is indicated. A peripherally located nucleus (N) is shown. (Reprinted with permission from Fawcett DW: A *Textbook of Histology*, 12th ed. New York, Chapman Hall, 1994, p 280. Courtesy of Don W. Fawcett, M.D.) (C–E). Electron micrographs of skeletal muscle cut in cross-section showing the characteristic arrangement of myofilaments in the H band, A band, and I band, respectively. The H band shows only thick myofilaments (*large black dots*). The A band shows both thick myofilaments (*large black dots*) surrounded by six thin myofilaments (*small black dots*). The I band shows only thin myofilaments (*small black dots*). (C and E reprinted with permission from Weiss L: *Histology: Cell and Tissue Biology*, 5th ed. New York, Elsevier, 1983, p 264. *D* reprinted with permission from Fawcett DW: A *Textbook of Histology*, 12th ed. New York, Chapman Hall, 1994, p 280. Courtesy of Don W. Fawcett, M.D.)

B. Neuromuscular junction (Figure 6-4; see I G)

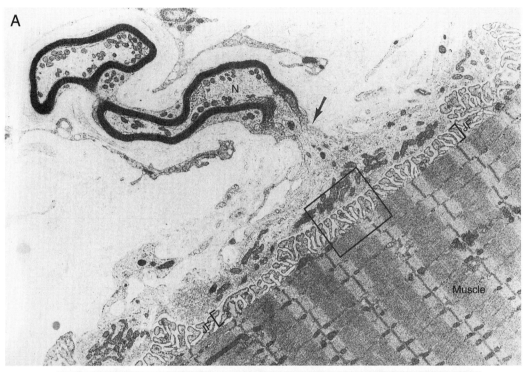

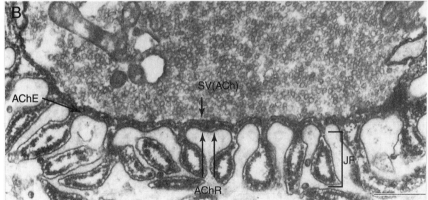

Figure 6-4. (A) Electron micrograph of a neuromuscular junction. A myelinated axon (N) loses its myelin sheath (at the *arrow*) and ends in a synaptic terminal on the surface of a skeletal muscle fiber (*muscle*). At the junction of the nerve and muscle fiber, the cell membrane of the muscle fiber is thrown into junctional folds (*jf; brackets*). The *boxed area* is shown at high magnification in B. (Reprinted with permission from Ellisman M: *J Cell Biol* 68:752, 1976.) (B) High magnification of the neuromuscular junction (*boxed area in A*). A collection of synaptic vesicles (*sv*) that contain acetylcholine (*ACh*) is indicated along with the presynaptic membrane (*single arrow*) where ACh is released. The postsynaptic membrane (*double arrows*) that contain ACh receptors (*AChR*) is shown. The *bracket* indicates the postsynaptic membrane of the skeletal muscle fiber thrown into junctional folds (*jf*). The synaptic cleft (*large arrow*) containing the electron-dense basal lamina and acetylcholinesterase (*AChE*) is shown. (Reprinted with permission from Lindgren CA, Emery DG, Haydon PG: Intracellular acidification reversibly reduces endocytosis at the neuromuscular junction. *J Neurosci* 17:3074, 1997.)

C. Intercalated disk (Figure 6-5; see II A 3)

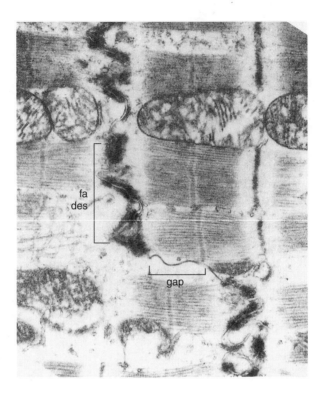

Figure 6-5.   Electron micrograph of an intercalated disk in cardiac muscle. An intercalated disk is found at the junction of two cardiac myocytes and is typically arranged in a stair-step pattern. The intercalated disk consists of a fascia adherens (*fa*), desmosomes (*des*), and gap junction (*gap*). The gap junction is always oriented parallel to the myofilaments. (Reprinted with permission from Wheater PR: *Functional Histology*. New York, Churchill Livingstone, 1987, p 94.)

7

Nervous Tissue

I. **THE NEURON** is the structural and functional unit of the nervous system. The neuron consists of a **perikaryon** (cell body), **dendrite,** and **axon,** each of which contains certain ultrastructural components (Table 7-1). The axon arises from an extension of the perikaryon called the **axon hillock.** The part of the axon between the axon hillock and the start of the myelin sheath is called the **initial segment** and is where the action potential is initiated.

   A. Axonal transport

   1. **Fast anterograde transport** is responsible for transporting **synaptic vesicles** from the perikaryon to the synaptic terminal and uses **kinesin,** which has adenosine triphosphatase (ATPase) activity.

   2. **Slow anterograde transport** is responsible for transporting **cytosol and cytoskeletal elements** from the perikaryon to the synaptic terminal.

   3. **Fast retrograde transport** is responsible for transporting **nerve growth factor, tetanus toxin, polio virus, rabies virus, and herpes simplex virus** from the synaptic terminal to the perikaryon and uses **dynein,** which has ATPase activity.

   B. Action potential (Figure 7-1)

   1. Within the neuronal **cytoplasm,** the sodium ion concentration is low and the potassium ion concentration is high. Within the **extracellular milieu,** the sodium ion concentration is high and the potassium ion concentration is low.

   2. Because of potassium ion leakage from the cytoplasm into the extracellular milieu and the Na^+-K^+-ATPase pump, a **resting membrane potential (-70 mV)** is established.

   3. When the membrane potential reaches **threshold (-55 mV),** an action potential occurs.

   4. At the peak of the action potential, the membrane potential reaches approximately **+50 mV** because of a **depolarization** due to an **influx of sodium ions.**

   5. At the nadir of the action potential, the membrane potential reaches approximately **-80 mV** because of a **hyperpolarization** due to an **efflux of potassium ions.**

   6. **Tetrodotoxin** (a poison found in puffer fish) and **saxitoxin** [a poison found in dinoflagellates ("red tides")] are potent sodium ion channel blockers.

   7. **Tetraethylammonium** (a poison) is a potent potassium ion channel blocker.

   C. Synapse (axodendritic)

   1. Synapses are areas of interaction between two neurons; for example, an axon and dendrite, forming an axodendritic synapse.

Table 7-1
Ultrastructural Components of Neuron

Cell Part	Ultrastructural Components
Perikaryon	Nucleus with prominent nucleolus, rER and polyribosomes (Nissl substance), Golgi complex, some sER, mitochondria, lysosomes, microfilaments (actin), neurofilaments (intermediate), microtubules, and inclusion bodies
Dendrite	Similar to perikaryon
Axon	Some sER, mitochondria, neurofilaments (intermediate), microtubules, and neurosecretory vesicles [rER, polyribosomes (Nissl substance), Golgi complex, and lysosomes are absent]

rER = rough endoplasmic reticulum; sER = smooth endoplasmic reticulum.

2. The **presynaptic membrane** of the axon releases the neurotransmitter.

3. The **postsynaptic membrane** of the dendrite has receptors for the neurotransmitter.

4. Binding of the neurotransmitter to receptor alters the conductance of the postsynaptic membrane to ions.

5. An influx of sodium ions **depolarizes** the postsynaptic neuron, producing an **excitatory postsynaptic potential (EPSP).**

6. An influx of chloride ions **hyperpolarizes** the postsynaptic neuron, producing an **inhibitory postsynaptic potential (IPSP).**

7. The EPSPs and IPSPs spread over the postsynaptic neuron by **electrotonic conduction.** If the momentary sum of the EPSPs and IPSPs reaches -55 mV (threshold), an action potential occurs at the **initial segment of the axon.** Note that an action potential does not occur at the synapse.

D. Node of Ranvier

    1. This is a segment of the axon exposed to the extracellular milieu due to gaps in the myelin sheath.

    2. It is the site where action potentials are **regenerated** due to the presence of **sodium ion channels.**

E. **Neurotransmitters** (Table 7-2)

F. **Fuel sources. Glucose** is the major fuel source for neurons. During starvation, **ketones** can be metabolized by neurons.

II. NEUROGLIAL CELLS are the nonneural cells of the nervous system.

A. **Oligodendrocytes** produce myelin in the central nervous system (CNS). One oligodendrocyte can myelinate several axons.

B. **Astrocytes** have the following characteristics and functions:

    1. Project foot processes to capillaries

    2. Play a role in the metabolism of neurotransmitters [e.g., glutamate, γ-aminobutyric acid (GABA), serotonin]

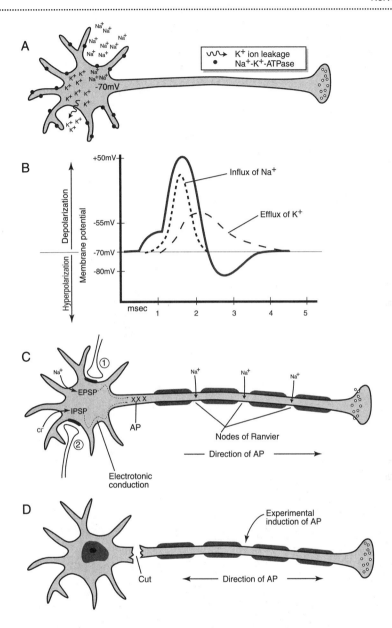

Figure 7-1. (A) Diagram depicting the sodium (Na$^+$) and potassium (K$^+$) ion concentrations in the neuron and extracellular milieu. (B) Diagram of an action potential. The influx of Na$^+$ (*thick dashed line*) and efflux of K$^+$ (*thin dashed line*) are indicated. (C) Synapse and generation of action potential. Two synapses (*1* and *2*) are shown. Synapse 1 allows for the influx of Na$^+$ (depolarization), causing an excitatory postsynaptic potential (*EPSP*). Synapse 2 allows for the influx of chloride ions (hyperpolarization), causing an inhibitory postsynaptic potential (*IPSP*). The EPSPs and IPSPs spread over the postsynaptic neuron by electrotonic conductance (*dotted lines*). If the sum reaches -55 mV (threshold), an action potential (*AP*) is generated at the initial segment of the axon. The AP is conducted along the axon and propagated, which means "new" APs are regenerated at the nodes of Ranvier due to an influx of sodium ions. (D) Diagram of a neuron cut so as to sever the perikaryon from the axon. If an AP is experimentally induced at mid-axon, the AP will be propagated along the axon in both directions; that is, toward both the perikaryon and synaptic terminal.

Table 7-2
Various Neurotransmitters

Neurotransmitter	Chemical Structure	Characteristics
Acetylcholine (ACh)	$CH_3-\overset{\displaystyle CH_3}{\underset{\displaystyle CH_3}{N}}-CH_2-CH_2O-\overset{O}{\underset{\parallel}{C}}-CH_3$	Uses the nicotinic ACh receptor (nAChR), which is a **transmitter-gated ion channel** that is permeable to Na^+, K^+, and Ca^{2+} ions Uses the muscarinic ACh receptor (mAChR), which is a **G protein-linked receptor** Is the neurotransmitter of the peripheral nervous system (PNS), neuromuscular junction, parasympathetic system, preganglionic sympathetic neurons, basal and visceral motor nuclei in the brain stem, and basal nucleus of Meynert (involved in Alzheimer's disease)
Catecholamines Epinephrine	$CH-CH_2-NH$ with OH and CH_3, HO, HO	Uses α_1, α_2, or β_1, β_2, β_3-adrenergic receptors, which are **G protein-linked receptors** Plays an insignificant role in the central nervous system (CNS) Is found in the adrenal medulla
Norepinephrine	$CH-CH_2-NH_2$ with OH, HO, HO	Uses α_1, α_2, or β_1, β_2, β_3-adrenergic receptors, which are **G protein-linked receptors** Is the transmitter of postganglionic sympathetic neurons and CNS (locus ceruleus) Plays a role in anxiety states, panic attacks, and depression
Dopamine	$CH_2-CH_2-NH_2$, HO, HO	Uses D1 and D2 dopamine receptors, which are **G protein-linked receptors** Is depleted in Parkinson disease Is increased in schizophrenia
Serotonin (5-hydroxy-tryptamine; 5-HT)	HO, $CH_2-CH_2-NH_2$, N	Uses the 5-HT receptor, which is a **transmitter-gated ion channel** that is permeable to Na^+ and K^+ ions Is the neurotransmitter of the raphe nuclei of the brain stem whose neurons project to widespread areas of the CNS
γ-Aminobutyric acid (GABA)	$H_2\overset{\displaystyle NH_2}{C}-CH_2-CH_2-COOH$	Uses the $GABA_A$ receptor, which is a **transmitter-gated ion channel** that is permeable to Cl^- ions Uses the $GABA_B$ receptor, which is a **G protein-linked receptor** Is the major **inhibitory** neurotransmitter of the CNS
Glycine	$H_3N-\overset{\displaystyle COOH}{\underset{\displaystyle H}{C}}-H$	Uses the glycine receptor, which is a **transmitter-gated ion channel** that is permeable to Cl^- ions Is the major **inhibitory** neurotransmitter of the spinal cord

(continued)

Table 7-2
Various Neurotransmitters

Neurotransmitter	Chemical Structure	Characteristics
Glutamate	$$COOH - \overset{\overset{\text{H}}{\mid}}{\underset{\underset{\text{NH}_2}{\mid}}{\text{C}}} - CH_2 - CH_2 - COOH$$	Uses the N-methyl-D-asparate (NMDA), kainate, or quisqualate A receptors, all of which are **transmitter-gated ion channels** that are permeable to Na^+, K^+, and Ca^{2+} ions Is the major **excitatory** neurotransmitter of the CNS
Opioid peptides		Use receptors that are **G protein-linked receptors**
Neuropeptides		Use receptors that are **G protein-linked receptors**

   3. Buffer the potassium ion concentration of the CNS extracellular space

   4. Form glial scars in a damaged area of the CNS (i.e., astrogliosis)

   5. Undergo hypertrophy and hyperplasia in reaction to CNS injury

   6. Contain the glial fibrillary acidic protein (GFAP)

  C. **Microglia** are derived from monocytes and have phagocytic function.

  D. **Ependymal cells** line the ventricles of the brain.

  E. **Tanycytes** are a modified type of ependymal cell that transports cerebrospinal fluid (CSF) to neurons in the hypothalamus.

  F. **Choroid epithelial cells** line the choroid plexus and produce CSF.

  G. **Schwann cells** produce myelin in the peripheral nervous system (PNS). One Schwann cell myelinates only one axon. Schwann cells invest all myelinated and unmyelinated axons of the PNS and are separated from each other by nodes of Ranvier.

III. THE BLOOD–BRAIN BARRIER

  A. The blood–brain barrier represents an anatomic and physiologic separation of blood from the CNS extracellular fluid.

  B. It consists of **tight junctions between nonfenestrated endothelial cells** with few pinocytic vesicles.

  C. It does not exist in some areas of the CNS, such as the median eminence, neurohypophysis, lamina terminalis, pineal gland, area postrema, and choroid plexus.

IV. THE BLOOD–CSF BARRIER consists of tight junctions between choroid epithelial cells of the choroid plexus.

V. NERVE DEGENERATION AND REGENERATION

  A. PNS

    1. **Degeneration. Anterograde (Wallerian) degeneration** of the axon and myelin sheath occurs distal to the site of injury. Macrophages infiltrate to remove cellular debris.

    a. **Chromatolysis** [loss of rough endoplasmic reticulum (rER)], movement of nucleus to the periphery, and hypertrophy of the perikaryon occurs.

    b. During this time, **muscle fasciculations** (small irregular contractions) occur caused by release of acetylcholine (ACh) from the degenerating synaptic terminal.

  2. Regeneration. Schwann cells proliferate and form a cord that is penetrated by the growing axon. The axon grows at 3 mm/day until it reaches the skeletal muscle.

    a. If the axon does not penetrate the cord of Schwann cells, the axon will not reach the skeletal muscle.

    b. During this time, **muscle fibrillations** (spontaneous repetitive contractions) occur caused by a supersensitivity of the muscle to ACh.

B. CNS

  1. Degeneration. Microglia phagocytose myelin and injured axons. Glial scars (astrogliosis) form.

  2. Regeneration. Effective regeneration does not occur in the CNS.

VI. CLINICAL CONSIDERATIONS

A. Huntington disease (HD) is an autosomal dominant mutation of the HD gene, which is located on the short (p) arm of chromosome 4 (i.e., **4p**) and encodes a protein called **Huntington.**

  1. The characteristic dysfunction is **cell death of cholinergic and GABA-ergic neurons** within the caudate nucleus. This results clinically in choreic (dance-like) movements, mood disturbances, and loss of mental activity.

  2. The mechanism for neuronal cell death may involve a **hyperactive glutamate receptor** [the N-methyl-D-aspartate (NMDA) receptor], resulting in **glutamate toxicity.**

  3. Glutamate toxicity results from an **excessive influx of calcium ions** into the neuron.

B. Parkinson disease is a degenerative disease that results in the **depletion of dopamine** and **loss of melanin-containing dopaminergic neurons** within the substantia nigra. This results clinically in bradykinesia, stooped posture, shuffling gait, and masked facies.

C. Motor neuron disease is a progressive disease caused by the death of motor neurons, the pathogenesis of which is not known.

  1. Death of upper motor neurons in the brain stem is called **progressive bulbar palsy.**

  2. Death of lower motor neurons in the spinal cord is called **progressive muscular atrophy.**

  3. Death of upper motor neurons of the corticospinal tract, corticobulbar tract, and brain stem, along with lower motor neurons of the spinal cord, is called **amyotrophic lateral sclerosis** (also called Lou Gehrig disease). Amyotrophic lateral sclerosis results clinically in hyperreflexia, spasticity, and Babinski reflex, along with muscle atrophy, weakness, and fasiculations.

D. Multiple sclerosis may be a type of autoimmune disease in which the myelin of the CNS is destroyed. This results clinically in paralysis, loss of sensation, and loss of coordination. The exact nature of the defect depends on the specific area of the CNS involved. Interferon beta-1a (Avonex) and interferon beta-1b (Betaseron) are used clinically to ameliorate the autoimmune attack on myelin.

E. Astrocytoma is a tumor of astrocytes that accounts for approximately 80% of adult primary brain tumors. Its hallmark is a proliferation of astrocytic cell processes of varying size that displace normal neurons. This results clinically in seizures, headaches, and focal neurologic deficits depending on the area of the CNS involved.

VII. SELECTED PHOTOMICROGRAPHS

A. Blood–brain barrier (Figure 7-2; see III)

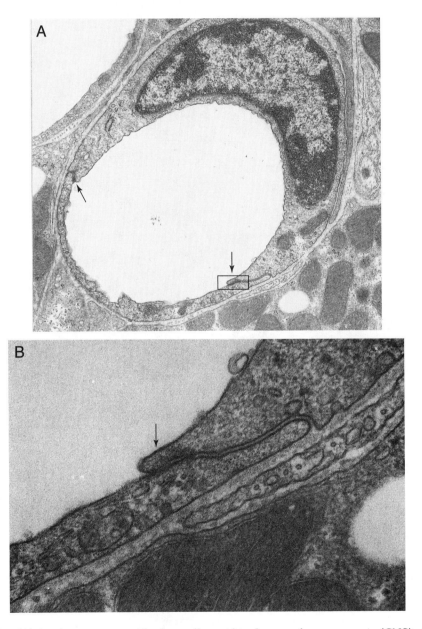

Figure 7-2.   (A) An electron micrograph of a capillary within the central nervous system (CNS). A zonula occludens (*arrows*) between two endothelial cells prevents the escape of macromolecules into the brain. This is the basis of the blood–brain barrier. A paucity of pinocytotic vesicles and astrocytic foot processes also may play a role in the barrier. (B) High magnification of the boxed area in A showing the zonula occludens (*arrow*) between two endothelial cells.

B. Oligodendrocyte (Figure 7-3; see II A)

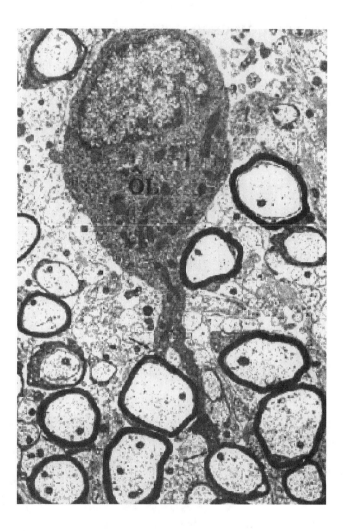

Figure 7-3. Electron micrograph of an oligodendrocyte (*OL*). Note the cell processes of the oligodendrocyte extending to two axons within the CNS and providing the myelin sheath. Note that one oligodendrocyte can myelinate several axons. (Reprinted with permission from Siegel GJ, Agranoff BW, Albers RW, et al: *Basic Neurochemistry*, 6th ed. Philadelphia, Lippincott-Raven, 1988, p 22.)

C. Node of Ranvier (Figure 7-4; see I D)

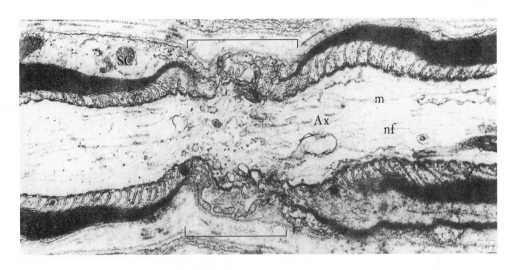

Figure 7-4. Electron micrograph of a longitudinal section of a myelinated axon of the adult sciatic nerve [i.e., peripheral nervous system (PNS)]. The myelin sheath in the PNS is formed by a Schwann cell (SC). The axon (Ax) with microtubules (m) and neurofilaments (nf) can be observed. The myelin sheath terminates at the node of Ranvier (*brackets*). The node of Ranvier is where action potentials are regenerated due to the presence of sodium ion channels that allow an influx of sodium ions to occur. (Reprinted with permission from Peters A, Palay SL, Webster HF: *The Fine Structure of the Nervous System: Neurons and Their Supporting Cells*, 3rd ed. London, Oxford University Press, 1990. © 1990 by Alan Peters. Used by permission of Oxford University Press, Inc.)

D. Synapse (Figure 7-5; see I C)

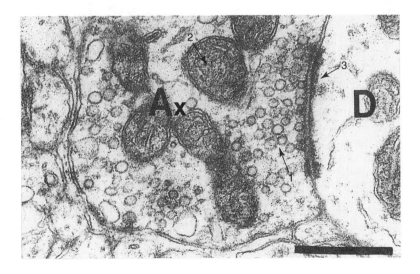

Figure 7-5. Electron micrograph of an axodendritic synapse [i.e., between an axon (Ax) and a dendrite (D)]. Synaptic vesicles (*arrow 1*), mitochondria (*arrow 2*), and a postsynaptic density (*arrow 3*) are identified. (Reprinted with permission from Chazel G, Baude A, Barbe A, et al: Ultrastructural organization of the interstitial subnucleus of the nucleus of the tractus solitarius in the cat: identification of vagal afferents. *J Neurocytol* 20:859, 1991.)

E. Myelinated and unmyelinated axons (Figure 7-6)

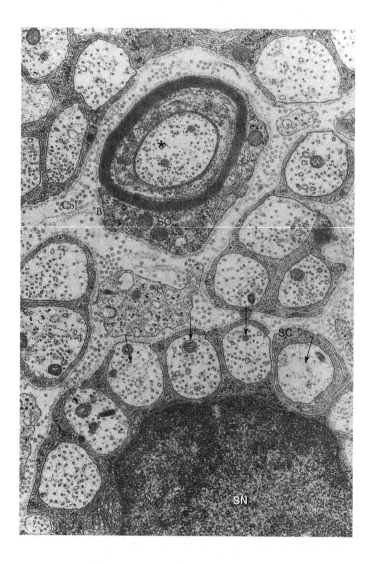

Figure 7-6. Electron micrograph of adult sciatic nerve (PNS) reveals a myelinated axon (*asterisk*) surrounded by a myelin sheath, Schwann cell cytoplasm, basal lamina (*B*), and collagen of the endoneurium (*Col*). Unmyelinated axons (*arrows*) are separately embedded within Schwann cell cytoplasm (*SC*) with no myelin sheath. *SN* = Schwann cell nucleus. (Reprinted with permission from Peters A, Palay SL, Webster HF: *The Fine Structure of the Nervous System: Neurons and Their Supporting Cells*, 3rd ed. London, Oxford University Press, 1990. © 1990 by Alan Peters. Used by permission of Oxford University Press, Inc.)

F. Astrocytoma (Figure 7-7; see VII E)

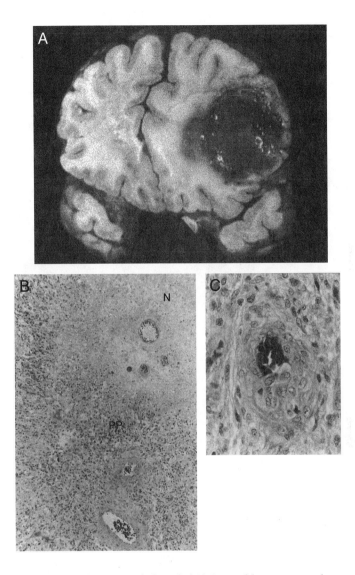

Figure 7-7. Astrocytoma (glioblastoma multiforme). (A) Coronal brain section shows a glioma in the left frontal cortex containing pigmentation due to hemorrhage. This 65-year-old woman demonstrated personality/behavioral changes during a period of several months. Her condition became increasingly more serious and eventually led to institutionalization for the last 2 weeks of her life. (Reprinted with permission from Woodard JS: *Complete Legend of Histologic Neuropathology Illustrations.* Orange, CA, California Medical Publications, 1982.) (B) Light micrograph indicating areas of necrosis (N) that are surrounded by areas of hypercellularity with highly anaplastic tumor cells crowded along the edges of the necrotic regions producing so-called pseudopalisading (PP). (Courtesy of the East Carolina University School of Medicine, Department of Pathology slide collection.) (C) Light micrograph of the vascular proliferation associated with astrocytoma. Tufts of endothelial may bulge into the vascular lumen with extreme examples forming glomeruloid structures. (Courtesy of the East Carolina University School of Medicine, Department of Pathology slide collection.)

G. Multiple sclerosis (Figure 7-8; see VII D)

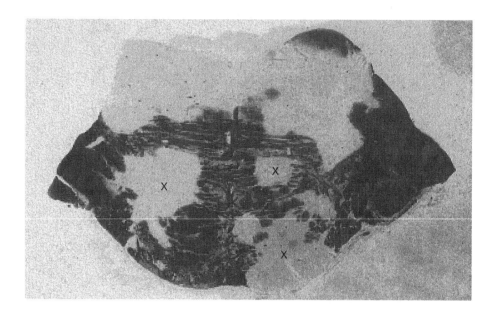

Figure 7-8. Multiple sclerosis. A cross-section through the pons is stained for myelin (black). Note the focal areas (X) where demyelination has occurred. (Reprinted with permission from Stevens A, Lowe J: *Human Histology,* 2nd ed. London, Mosby, 1997, p 87.)

8

Heart and Blood Vessels

I. HEART LAYERS

A. Endocardium

    1. Endocardium is lined by endothelium.

    2. It is underlain by the **subendocardial layer,** which contains blood vessels, nerves, and Purkinje myocytes.

    3. It is continuous with the tunica intima of blood vessels.

B. Myocardium consists of the following cell types:

    1. Cardiac myocytes (see Chapter 6 II A)

        a. Cardiac myocytes contract through intrinsically generated action potentials, which are then passed on to neighboring myocytes by gap junctions; that is, the heart beat is myogenic.

        b. The action potentials are generated by ion fluxes in the cardiac myocytes (Figure 8-1), and can be divided into phases:

           (1) Phase 0 is due to the **influx of sodium ions** into the cardiac myocyte through **fast sodium channels. Tetrodotoxin** and many drugs that treat cardiac arrhythmias block fast sodium channels.

           (2) Phase 1 is due to a brief efflux of potassium ions through potassium channels, which can be blocked by **4-aminopyridine.**

           (3) Phase 2 is due to the **influx of calcium ions** into the cardiac myocyte through **L-type calcium channels** located on the cell membrane and T tubule. This influx of calcium ions is involved in contraction of cardiac myocytes. **Verapamil** and **diltiazem** block calcium channels, thereby reducing the strength of contraction. However, these drugs are used in patients with congestive heart failure (CHF) to inhibit vascular smooth muscle contraction, causing vasodilation (not because of their effect on cardiac myocytes). The peripheral vasodilation reduces the load on the heart. These drugs are often referred to as **afterload-reducing drugs.**

           (4) Phase 3 is due to an efflux of potassium ions that is greater than the influx of calcium ions.

           (5) Phase 4 is due to **removal of the excess sodium ions** that entered in phase 0 by Na^+–K^+–adenosine triphosphatase (ATPase) and **removal of the excess calcium ions** that entered in phase 2 by the Na^+/Ca^{2+} **exchanger. Cardiac glycosides** (e.g., **digitalis, ouabain**) block $Na+$–$K+$–ATPase, thereby elevating intracellular sodium level. The elevated sodium level overwhelms the Na^+/Ca^{2+} exchanger so that more calcium ions can be reaccumulated by terminal cisternae (TC). During the next contraction,

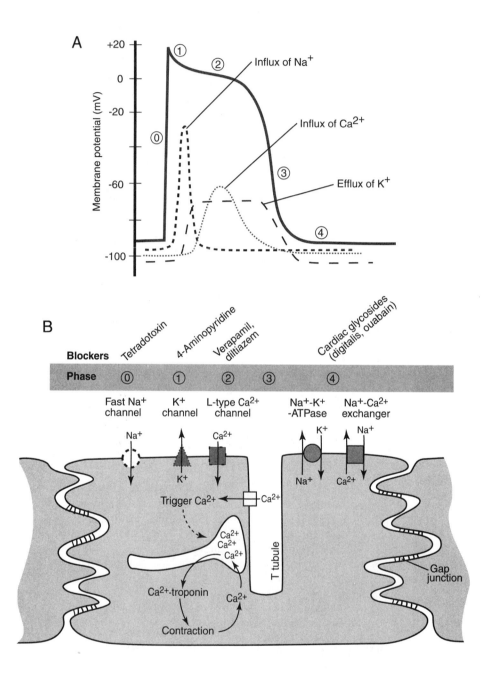

Figure 8-1. (A) Phases of the action potential generated by cardiac myocytes and pattern of sodium (Na^+), potassium (K^+), and calcium (Ca^{2+}) ion fluxes. (B) The ion fluxes are mediated by various ion channels in the cell membrane and T tubule of the cardiac myocyte. The influx of Ca^{2+} in phase 2 acts as trigger calcium that stimulates the release of a large pool of Ca^{2+} from the terminal cisternae. This leads to cardiac myocyte contraction. Various drugs are indicated that act as blockers of specific ion channels.

more calcium ions are released from TC, increasing the strength of contraction. Cardiac glycosides are used in patients with CHF to increase the strength of contraction.

2. Purkinje myocytes are modified cardiac myocytes that are specialized for conduction. Purkinje myocytes are *not* neurons. They are joined by gap junctions.

3. Myocardial endocrine cells are found in the right and left atria and have secretory granules containing **atrial natriuretic peptide (ANP).**

   a. ANP is secreted in response to increased blood volume or increased venous pressure within the atria (e.g., atrial distention due to left atrial failure).

   b. ANP functions

     (1) ANP increases glomerular filtration pressure and glomerular filtration rate (via vasoconstriction of the efferent arteriole) and decreases sodium resorption by the proximal convoluted tubule (PCT). These actions produce **natriuresis** (increased sodium excretion) in a large volume of dilute urine.

     (2) ANP inhibits secretion of **antidiuretic hormone (ADH)** from the neurohypophysis.

     (3) ANP inhibits secretion of **aldosterone** from the adrenal cortex (zona glomerulosa).

     (4) ANP inhibits secretion of **renin** from juxtaglomerular cells.

     (5) ANP causes vasodilation of peripheral and renal blood vessels.

C. Epicardium consists of connective tissue and a layer of mesothelium. In gross anatomy, the epicardium is called the visceral layer of the pericardial sac.

II. CONTRACTION OF CARDIAC MYOCYTES (Figure 8-1)

A. A diad consists of a T tubule located at the Z disk and flanked by one terminal cisterna. A T tubule is an invagination of the cell membrane. TC are dilated sacs of sarcoplasmic reticulum that store, release, and reaccumulate calcium ions.

B. The influx of calcium ions that occurs at the cell membrane and T tubule in phase 2 of the action potential is not sufficient to cause contraction, but acts as **trigger calcium,** which stimulates the release of a large pool of calcium ions stored in TC.

C. Calcium ions bind to troponin, which allows the **myosin cross-bridge—ADP—PO$_4^{2-}$** complex to bind to actin (see Figure 6-2).

D. ADP–PO$_4^{2-}$ is released, leaving the myosin cross-bridge bound to actin.

E. The myosin cross-bridge binds ATP, which detaches the myosin cross-bridge from actin.

F. ATP is hydrolyzed by myosin ATPase, and the products (ADP and PO$_4^{2-}$) remain bound to the myosin cross-bridge, thereby reforming the myosin cross-bridge—ADP—PO$_4^{2-}$ complex.

G. As the influx of calcium ions begins to decrease at the end of phase 2, TC reaccumulate calcium ions.

H. Troponin is freed of calcium ions.

III. CONDUCTION SYSTEM (Figure 8-2)

A. The sinoatrial (SA) node is the pacemaker of the heart. It is located at the junction of the superior vena cava and the right atrium.

   1. Phase 0 of the action potential generated by the SA node is not produced by an influx of sodium ions, and is therefore not sensitive to tetrodotoxin.

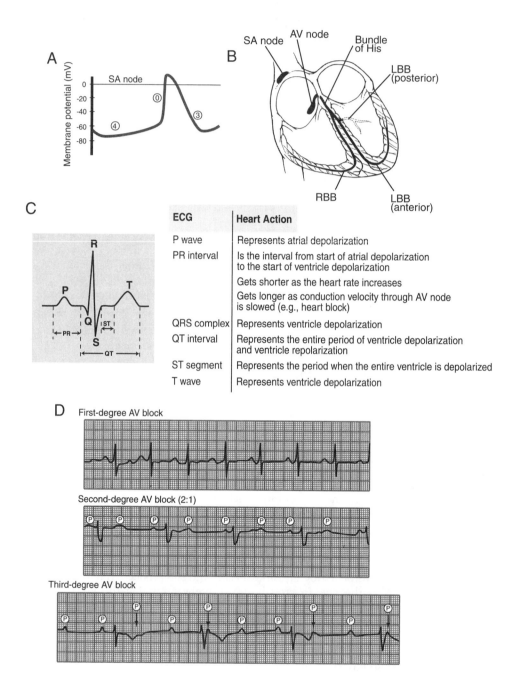

ECG	Heart Action
P wave	Represents atrial depolarization
PR interval	Is the interval from start of atrial depolarization to the start of ventricle depolarization
	Gets shorter as the heart rate increases
	Gets longer as conduction velocity through AV node is slowed (e.g., heart block)
QRS complex	Represents ventricle depolarization
QT interval	Represents the entire period of ventricle depolarization and ventricle repolarization
ST segment	Represents the period when the entire ventricle is depolarized
T wave	Represents ventricle depolarization

Figure 8-2. (A) The action potential generated by the sinoatrial (SA) node consisting of phases 4, 0, and 3. Compare this action potential with action potential of cardiac myocytes in Figure 8-1(A). (B) A diagram of the heart conduction system. (C) Normal electrocardiogram measured from lead II and *table* of the heart actions. (D) Electrocardiogram of first-degree heart block in which the PR interval is 0.28 seconds (> 0.20 seconds is abnormal). Electrocardiogram of second-degree heart block in which all QRS complexes are preceded by P waves, but not all P waves are followed by QRS complexes. Electrocardiogram of third-degree heart block in which P waves and QRS complexes are disassociated. (Reprinted with permission from Berne RM, Levy MN: *Physiology*, 4th ed. St. Louis, Mosby, 1998, p 355.) *AV* = atrioventricular node; *LBB* = left bundle branch; *RBB* = right bundle branch; *SA* = sinoatrial node.

2. Phase 4 of the action potential generated by the SA node is a slow diastolic depolarization that proceeds until threshold is reached.

3. From the SA node, the impulse spreads throughout the right atrium to the left atrium, and eventually to the atrioventricular (AV) node.

4. **Ectopic pacemakers** are present in the normal heart, and their added activity may induce continuous rhythm disturbances, such as **paroxysmal tachycardias.** When the ectopic pacemaker stops functioning, the SA node may remain quiescent for a period of time (called **SA node recovery time**). In patients with **sick sinus syndrome,** the SA node recovery time is prolonged with a period of asystole (absence of heartbeat) and loss of consciousness.

5. If all SA node activity is destroyed, the AV node assumes the pacemaker role.

B. **The AV node** is located on the right side of the interatrial septum near the ostium of the coronary sinus.

1. The delay between the start of the **P wave** (atrial depolarization) and the **QRS complex** (ventricle depolarization) occurs at the AV node. This normal delay allows for optimal ventricular filling during atrial contraction.

2. A **first-degree heart block** occurs when there is an abnormally long delay at the AV node.

C. AV conduction

1. A **second-degree heart block** occurs when only a portion of atrial impulses are conducted to the ventricles.

2. A **third-degree heart block** occurs when no atrial impulses are conducted to the ventricles.

3. **Wolff-Parkinson-White syndrome** is a congenital disorder in which an **accessory conduction pathway** between the atria and ventricles exists. This syndrome is ordinarily asymptomatic. However, a re-entry loop may develop in which impulses travel to the ventricles via the normal conduction pathway but return to the atria via the accessory pathway, causing **supraventricular tachycardia.**

D. Bundle of His, bundle branches, and Purkinje myocytes

1. The **bundle of His** travels in the subendocardial layer on the right side of the interventricular septum.

2. It divides into **right and left bundle branches.** The left bundle branch further divides into a thin anterior division and a thick posterior division.

3. The right and left bundle branches terminate in a complex network of the **Purkinje myocytes.**

IV. NEURAL REGULATION OF HEART RATE. The autonomic nervous system modulates the myogenic heartbeat.

A. **The parasympathetic system** decreases the heart rate.

1. The cell bodies of preganglionic neurons are located in the **dorsal nucleus of the vagus** and **nucleus ambiguus** of the medulla. The axons of preganglionic neurons run in the vagus (X) nerve and use acetylcholine (ACh) as a neurotransmitter.

2. The cell bodies of postganglionic neurons are located near the **SA node and AV conduction tissue.** The axons of postganglionic neurons terminate on the SA node and AV conduction tissue and use ACh as a neurotransmitter.

3. ACh binds to the **muscarinic ACh receptor (mAChR),** which is a G protein-linked receptor that inhibits adenylate cyclase and decreases cyclic adenosine monophosphate (cAMP) levels.

4. The SA node and AV conduction tissue contain high levels of **acetylcholinesterase** (degrades ACh rapidly) such that any given vagal stimulation is **short-lived.**

5. Atropine is an mAChR antagonist; therefore, atropine increases the heart rate.

6. Vasovagal syncope is a brief period of lightheadedness or loss of consciousness due to an intense burst of vagus (X) nerve activity that decreases the heart rate.

B. The **sympathetic system** increases the heart rate.

1. The cell bodies of preganglionic neurons are located in the **intermediolateral columns** of the spinal cord. The axons of preganglionic neurons enter the paravertebral ganglion and travel to the stellate/middle cervical ganglia and use ACh as a neurotransmitter.

2. The cell bodies of postganglionic neurons are located in the **stellate and middle cervical ganglia.** The axons of postganglionic neurons are distributed to the myocardium-accompanying blood vessels and use norepinephrine (NE) as a neurotransmitter.

3. NE binds to **β-adrenergic receptors,** which are G protein-linked receptors that stimulate adenylate cyclase and increase cAMP levels. Consequently, protein kinases are activated, which promotes phosphorylation of various proteins that activate calcium channels of the cardiac myocytes to increase the influx of calcium ions.

4. Released NE either is carried away by the bloodstream or is taken up by the nerve terminals so that sympathetic stimulation is relatively **long-lived.**

5. Propranolol is a β-adrenergic antagonist; therefore, propranolol decreases the heart rate.

V. ENZYME LEVELS IN MYOCARDIAL INFARCTION (Table 8-1). Creatine kinase

(CK) and lactate dehydrogenase (LDH) serum isoenzyme levels are useful in diagnosing myocardial infarction. These isoenzymes normally are confined to the cytoplasm of cardiac myocytes; however, ischemia allows for the leakage of these isoenzymes into the serum. Isoenzymes catalyze the same reaction but have different amino acid sequences and properties.

A. CK levels. CK consists of M and B subunits. CK-1 (MM subunits) is found in skeletal muscle and cardiac muscle. CK-2 (MB subunits) is found in cardiac muscle. CK-3 (BB subunits) is found in brain. **An elevated total CK-1 and CK-2 fraction** provides early confirmation of myocardial infarction.

B. LDH levels. LDH consists of H and M subunits. LDH_1 (HHHH subunits) is found in cardiac muscle and red blood cells. LDH_2 (HHHM subunits) is found in cardiac muscle and red blood cells. LDH_3 (HHMM subunits) is found in brain and kidney. LDH4 (HMMM subunits) is found in liver and skeletal muscle. LDH_5 (MMMM subunits) is found in liver and skeletal muscle. A **reversed LDH_1:LDH_2 ratio** at 24 hours after admission is a characteristic sign for confirmation of myocardial infarction.

VI. BLOOD VESSELS

A. Tunics

1. Tunica intima consists of endothelium, a basal lamina, loose connective tissue, and an internal elastic lamina.

Table 8-1

Changes in Creatine Kinase and Lactate Dehydrogenase Serum Levels in Myocardial Infarction

Time	CK Total	CK-2 Fraction	LDH
Admission	180 U/L	7%	N/A
12 hours after admission	230 U/L	8%	N/A
24 hours after admission	290 U/L	10%	
Normal values	30–170 U/L	<5%	

U/L = units/liter; CK = creatine kinase; LDH = lactate dehydrogenase; N/A = not applicable.

2. **Tunica media** consists of smooth muscle cells, type III collagen, elastic fibers, and an external elastic lamina.

3. **Tunica adventitia** consists of fibroblasts, type I collagen, and some elastic fibers.

B. Elastic (conducting) arteries (e.g., pulmonary artery, aorta) have a tunica media with a prominent elastic fiber component that responds to the high systolic pressure generated by the heart.

C. Muscular (distributing) arteries have a tunica intima with a prominent internal elastic lamina and a tunica media with a prominent smooth muscle cell component.

D. Arterioles have a tunica media that consists of only one to two layers of smooth muscle cells and play a major role in regulation of blood pressure. **Metarterioles** are the smallest (or terminal) branches of the arterial system and play a role in regulation of blood flow to capillary beds.

E. Arteriovenous anastomoses (AVA) allow arteriolar blood to bypass the capillary bed and empty directly into venules. AVA are found primarily in the skin to regulate body temperature. Constriction of the arteriolar component directs blood to the capillary bed causing depletion of body heat. Dilation of the arteriolar component directs blood to the venules causing conservation of body heat.

F. Capillaries consist of a single layer of endothelial cells surrounded by a basal lamina and are the site of exchange (e.g., CO_2, O_2, nutrients) between blood and cells. Microvasculature damage associated with type 1 and type 2 diabetes is due to **nonenzymatic glycosylation** of various proteins, which causes the release of harmful cytokines. The different types of capillaries include the following:

1. **Continuous capillaries** consist of a single layer of endothelial cells joined by a zonula occludens (tight junction) and contain no fenestrae (or pores). They are found in lung, muscle, and brain.

2. **Fenestrated capillaries** consist of a single layer of endothelial cells joined by a zonula occludens (tight junction) and contain fenestrae (or pores) with diaphragms. They are found in endocrine glands, intestine, and kidney. Fenestrated capillaries without diaphragms are found solely within the kidney glomerulus.

3. **Discontinuous capillaries (sinusoids)** consist of a single layer of endothelial cells that are separated by wide gaps (i.e., no zonula occludens present) and contain fenestrae. They are found in the liver, bone marrow, and spleen.

VII. FUNCTIONS OF ENDOTHELIUM

A. **Secretion** of the following substances:

1. **von Willebrand factor** is stored in Weibel-Palade granules and promotes platelet adhesion to subendothelial collagen at an injury site, as well as blood coagulation. von Willebrand disease is a common bleeding disorder in humans.

2. **Nitric oxide (NO)** affects smooth muscle cells of the tunica media and causes vasodilation.

   a. NO is synthesized by the reaction:

   $$\text{Arginine} \xrightarrow{\text{NO synthase}} \text{NO} + \text{Citrulline}$$

   b. NO activates guanylate cyclase in smooth muscle cells, causing **increased levels of cyclic guanosine monophosphate (cGMP)** and **vasodilation.**

   c. NO is involved in the vasodilation associated with penile erection. **Viagra** used in the treatment of erectile dysfunction is a **cGMP phosphodiesterase inhibitor.** With its use, increased cGMP levels are maintained.

   d. The vasodilation effects of **nitroglycerin** and **amyl nitrates** occur through their conversion to NO.

3. **Prostacyclin (PGI$_2$)** causes vasodilation and inhibits platelet aggregation. PGI$_2$ is synthesized from arachidonic acid using the enzymes cyclooxygenase and PGI synthase.

4. **Endothelin 1** affects smooth muscle cells of the tunica media and causes vasoconstriction.

B. **Conversion** of the following substances:

1. **Angiotensin I to angiotensin II,** which causes vasoconstriction and secretion of both aldosterone and ADH

2. Bradykinin, serotonin, norepinephrine, prostaglandins, and thrombin to inert compounds

C. **Breakdown** of lipoproteins to triglycerides and cholesterol

VIII. BLOOD FLOW

A. **Modification.** Blood flow to an organ is modified in a number of ways.

1. **Autoregulation** is the phenomenon whereby blood flow to an organ remains constant over a wide range of pressures.

2. **Active hyperemia** is the phenomenon whereby blood flow to an organ is proportional to its metabolic activity.

3. **Reactive hyperemia** is the phenomenon whereby blood flow to an organ is increased after a period of occlusion.

B. **Modification theories.** Modification of blood flow to an organ is explained by the following:

1. The **metabolic hypothesis** states that vasodilator metabolites are released upon an increase in tissue activity.

2. The **myogenic hypothesis** states that vascular smooth muscle contracts upon stretching.

IX. TYPES OF CIRCULATION (Table 8-2)

Table 8-2
Types of Circulation

Circulation	Percent of Cardiac Output	Blood Flow Demonstrates	Control
Coronary	5	Autoregulation Active hyperemia Reactive hyperemia	Hypoxia and adenosine cause vasodilation
Cerebral	15	Autoregulation Active hyperemia Reactive hyperemia	Increased Pco_2 or decreased pH cause vasodilation
Skeletal muscle	20	Autoregulation Active hyperemia Reactive hyperemia	During exercise, lactate, adenosine, and K^+ cause vasodilation At rest, sympathetic innervation through NE release stimulates α-adrenergic receptors, causing vasoconstriction At rest, sympathetic innervation through NE release stimulates β-adrenergic receptors, causing vasodilation
Kidney	25	Autoregulation	Renal blood flow remains constant from 100–200 mm Hg arterial pressure.
Respiratory	100	Hypoxic vasoconstriction	Hypoxia causes vasoconstriction so that blood is directed away from poorly ventilated areas to well-ventilated areas of the lung It is the only circulation that responds to hypoxia by vasoconstriction
Skin	5	Temperature regulation	Increase the temperature: sympathetic innervation causes vasodilation, directing blood to the surface

NE = norepinephrine.

X. SELECTED PHOTOMICROGRAPHS

A. Normal muscular artery (Figure 8-3; see VI C)

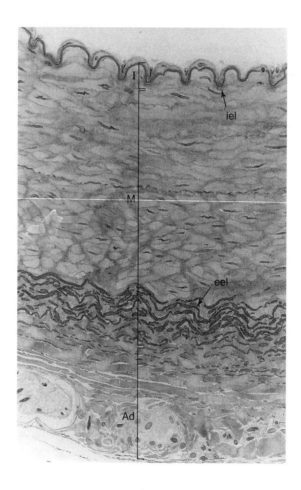

Figure 8-3. Light micrograph of a muscular artery. The tunica intima (*I*), tunica media (*M*), and tunica adventitia (*Ad*) are indicated. *eel* = external elastic lamina; *iel* = internal elastic lamina.

B. Coronary artery atherosclerosis (Figure 8-4)

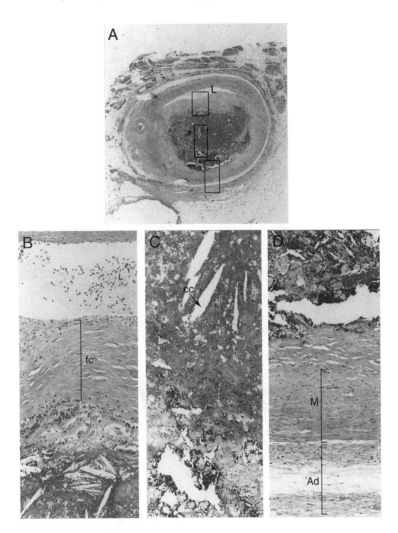

Figure 8-4. (A) Coronary artery with atherosclerosis. The entire coronary artery is shown with a eccentric, narrow lumen (L) due to the presence of an atheromatous plaque (tunica intima thickening). Atherosclerosis is considered an **intimal disease.** (B, C, D) High magnification of the *boxed areas* (shown in A) of the atheromatous plaque. The fibrous cap (*fc*) is composed of smooth muscle cells, a few leukocytes, and a relatively dense deposition of collagen. The deeper necrotic core (see C) consists of a disorganized mass of lipid material, cholesterol crystals (*cc*), cell debris, and foam cells. Ad = tunica adventitia; M = tunica media. [An atheromatous plaque may undergo many histologic changes, such as: (1) **calcification** that turns arteries into brittle pipes, (2) **hemorrhage** into the plaque that occurs and induces focal rupture of ulceration, (3) focal rupture at the luminal surface that results in **thrombus formation,** whereby the thrombus may partially or completely occlude the lumen, leading to approximately 90% of all myocardial infarctions. In this situation, thrombus formation is initiated by platelet aggregation induced by **thromboxane (TXA$_2$).** TXA$_2$ is synthesized from arachidonic acid using the enzyme cyclooxygenase. **Aspirin** covalently inhibits cyclooxygenase, and **nonsteroidal anti-inflammatory drugs (NSAIDs)** such as **ibuprofen and acetaminophen** reversibly inhibit cyclooxygenase and thereby block the synthesis of TXA$_2$. Consequently, low doses of aspirin and NSAIDs are effective in prevention of myocardial infarction. Thrombolysis is stimulated by **tissue plasminogen activator (TPA)** treatment, which successfully decreases the extent of ischemic damage due to myocardial infarction. TPA stimulates the **conversion of plasminogen to plasmin.** Plasmin is a protease that digests fibrin within the thrombus.] (Reprinted with permission from East Carolina University, School of Medicine, Department of Pathology slide collection.)

C. Myocardial infarction (Figure 8-5; see V)

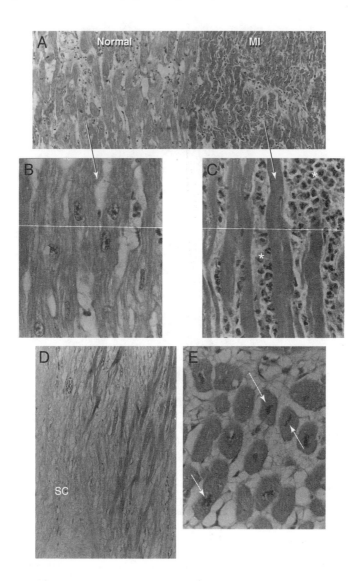

Figure 8-5. Myocardial infarction. (A) Low magnification of the myocardium (24–36 hours after ischemia) showing normal (undamaged) cardiac myocytes and damaged cardiac myocytes (*MI*). (B) High magnification of normal cardiac myocytes, which are relatively straight with some branching and contain a centrally located nucleus and very little intercellular space. (C) High magnification of damaged cardiac myocytes, which show the following characteristics: wavy appearance, no conspicuous nucleus, loss of striations, and an intercellular space filled with inflammatory exudate (*) composed mostly of neutrophils. The necrosis associated with myocardial infarction begins in the myocardium closest to the endocardium. (*D, E*) Old myocardial infarction. The damaged cardiac myocytes are replaced with collagenous scar tissue (*sc*). The cardiac myocytes adjacent to the scar represent a compensatory hypertrophy. These myocytes usually show bizarre-shaped nuclei, as indicated in *E* (cross-section of cardiac myocytes). (Reprinted with permission from the East Carolina University, School of Medicine, Department of Pathology slide collection.)

D. Purkinje myocyte (Figure 8-6; see III D 3)

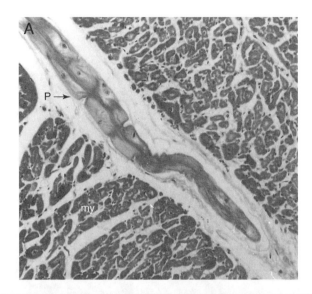

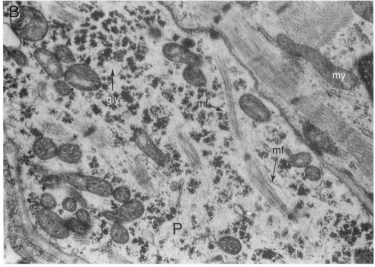

Figure 8-6.   Purkinje cell. (A) Light micrograph of Purkinje cells (P) traveling within the myocardium (my). By light microscopy, Purkinje cells appear pale because the large amount of glycogen that is normally contained in the cytoplasm is lost during histologic processing. (B) Electron micrograph of a Purkinje cell (P) showing large amount of glycogen (gly) and few myofilaments (mf). A portion of a cardiac myocyte within the myocardium (my) is also shown. (Courtesy of Dr. S. Viragh, Postgraduate Medical School, Budapest, Hungary.)

E. Fenestrated capillary with diaphragm (Figure 8-7; see VI F 2)

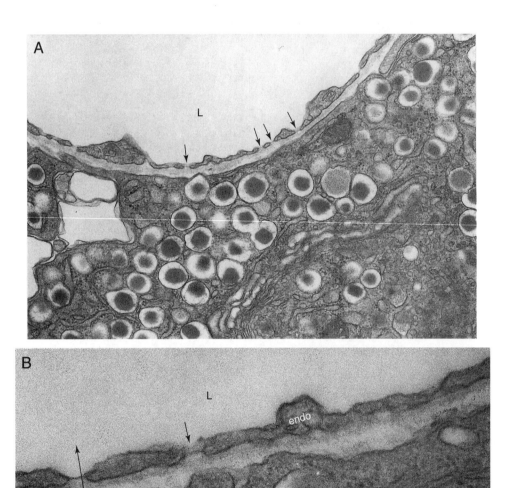

Figure 8-7.   Fenestrated capillary with diaphragms. (A) Low-magnification electron micrograph of a fenestrated capillary within the pancreatic islets of Langerhans (an endocrine gland) adjacent to a beta cell. The fenestrae with diaphragms are indicated at the *arrows*. L = lumen of the capillary. (B) High-magnification electron micrograph of a fenestrated capillary showing insulin (*I*) within a secretory granule and its route of release through the fenestrae (*large arrow*) into the lumen (L) of the capillary. The *small arrow* indicates fenestrae with diaphragm. *endo* = endothelial cell.

F. Kaposi sarcoma (Figure 8-8)

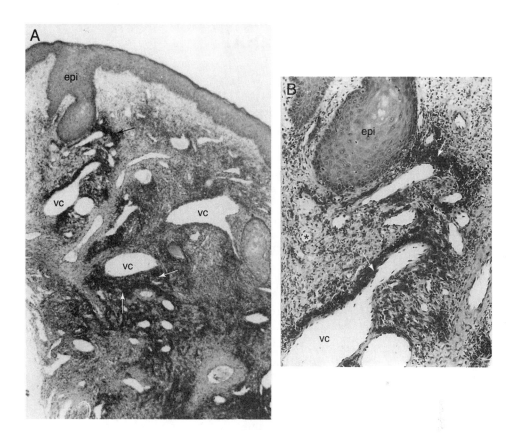

Figure 8-8.   Kaposi sarcoma. Kaposi sarcoma is a relatively rare vascular tumor but has come to the forefront because of its high frequency of occurrence in AIDS patients. Multiple red-to-purple skin plaques are observed clinically. (A,B) Low- and high-magnification light micrographs show an intact epidermis (*epi*) of the skin covering the malignant vascular lesion in the dermis consisting of numerous vascular channels (*vc*), spindle-shaped neoplastic stromal cells (*), and extravasated red blood cells (*arrows*). (Reprinted with permission from the East Carolina University, School of Medicine, Department of Pathology slide collection.)

9
Blood

I. PLASMA is the fluid portion of blood that contains many different proteins, such as **albumin,** which maintains blood colloidal osmotic (oncotic) pressure; **gamma globulins; beta globulins,** which participate in the transport of hormones, metal ions, and lipids; and **fibrinogen,** which participates in blood clotting. Plasma without fibrinogen is called **serum.**

II. RED BLOOD CELLS (RBCs or erythrocytes)

    A. Characteristics

        1. RBCs do not contain a nucleus or mitochondria.

        2. RBCs use **glucose** as the primary fuel source (i.e., **glycolysis** or **hexose monophosphate shunt** during stress).

        3. RBCs are biconcave-shaped disks (shape maintained by spectrin) and contain both **hemoglobin** and **carbonic anhydrase.**

    B. Layers. If blood is centrifuged (and clotting is prevented), three layers are separated:

        1. Top layer: plasma

        2. Middle layer: **buffy coat** containing **leukocytes** and **platelets**

        3. Bottom layer: RBCs

    C. Hematocrit is the percent volume of a blood sample occupied by RBCs. A normal hematocrit value is **45%.** Hematocrit values less than 45% may indicate **anemia.**

    D. Environment

        1. A **hypotonic** environment causes RBCs to swell, rupture (thereby forming ghosts), and release hemoglobin. This process is called **hemolysis.**

        2. A **hypertonic** environment causes RBCs to shrink so that spiny projections protrude from the surface. This process is called **crenation.**

    E. Blood group antigens. The A, B, and O blood group antigens are **carbohydrates** linked to lipids of the RBC membrane. Because these carbohydrate antigens are genetically determined, an individual who receives mismatched blood will mount an immune reaction.

        1. Type O blood is the universal **donor.**

        2. Type AB blood is the universal **recipient.**

    F. The **Rh factor** is clinically important in pregnancy. If the mother is Rh−, she will produce Rh antibodies if the fetus is Rh+. This situation will not affect the first pregnancy, but will affect the second pregnancy with an Rh+ fetus.

1. In the second pregnancy with an Rh+ fetus, a hemolytic condition of RBCs occurs known as **erythroblastosis fetalis.**

2. Kernicterus, which is a pathologic deposition of bilirubin in the basal ganglia, may develop due to the jaundice from the RBC hemolysis.

III. HEMOGLOBIN (Hb)

A. Characteristics

1. Hb is a **globular protein** consisting of **four subunits.**
  a. Adult Hb (HbA) consists of two alpha-globin subunits and two beta-globin subunits designated **Hb $\alpha_2\beta_2$.**
  b. Fetal Hb (HbF) consists of two alpha-globin subunits and two gamma-globin subunits designated **Hb $\alpha_2\gamma_2$.** HbF is the major form of Hb during **pregnancy** because the oxygen affinity of HbF is higher than the oxygen affinity of HbA and thereby pulls oxygen from the maternal blood into fetal blood. The higher oxygen affinity of HbF is explained by **2,3-bisphosphoglycerate (BPG).** When 2,3-BPG binds HbA, the oxygen affinity of HbA is lowered. However, 2,3-BPG does not bind HbF, and therefore, **the oxygen affinity of HbF is higher.**

2. Hb contains a **heme** moiety, which is an **iron (Fe)-containing porphyrin.** Fe^{2+} (ferrous state) binds oxygen, forming **oxyhemoglobin.** Fe^{3+} (ferric state) does not bind oxygen, forming **deoxyhemoglobin.** The heme moiety is synthesized partially in mitochondria and partially in cytoplasm.

3. The **Hb–O_2 dissociation curve** is **sigmoid** shaped because each successive oxygen that binds to Hb increases the affinity for the next oxygen (i.e., binding is cooperative). Therefore, the affinity for the fourth oxygen is the highest.

4. Concentration of Hb
  a. In **men and boys,** the concentration of Hb is **15 g/100 ml blood.**
  b. In **women and girls,** the concentration of Hb is **13.5 g/100 ml blood.**

B. Clinical considerations

1. Thalassemia syndromes are a heterogeneous group of genetic defects characterized by the lack of or decreased synthesis of either α-globin (α-thalassemia) or β-globin (β-thalassemia).
  a. Hydrops fetalis is the most severe form of α-thalassemia and causes severe pallor, generalized edema, and massive hepatosplenomegaly, and invariably leads to intrauterine fetal death.
  b. β-Thalassemia major is the most severe form of β-thalassemia and causes a severe, transfusion-dependent anemia. It is most common in Mediterranean countries and parts of Africa and southeast Asia.

2. Types 1 and 2 diabetes. The amount of **glycosylated Hb** is an indicator of blood glucose normalization over the previous 3 months (because the half-life of RBCs is 3 months) in patients with type 1 and type 2 diabetes. Long periods of elevated blood glucose levels result in a glycosylated Hb (i.e., HbA_{1c}) of 12%–20%, whereas normal levels are approximately 5%.

IV. BLOOD GAS EXCHANGE (Figure 9-1)

A. Characteristics

1. Oxygen is not soluble in plasma, so it is transported by Hb.

2. Approximately 90% of CO_2 is transported as HCO_3^- in plasma.

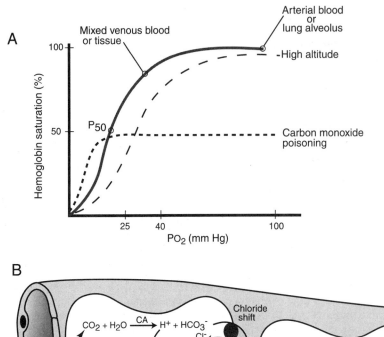

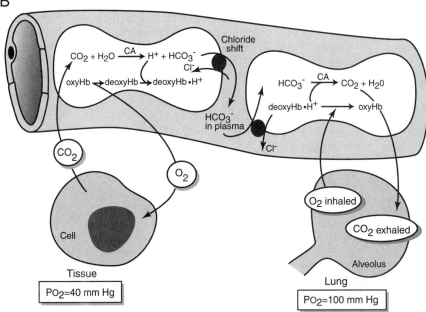

Figure 9-1. (A) Hemoglobin (Hb)–oxygen (O_2) dissociation curve. Note the sigmoid shape of the curve. At a PO_2 of 100 mm Hg found in arterial blood and lung alveoli, Hb is 100% saturated. At a PO_2 of 40 mm Hg found in mixed venous blood and tissues, Hb is 75% saturated. At a PO_2 of 25 mm Hg, Hb is 50% saturated (P_{50}). At high altitudes, the curve is shifted to the right, which facilitates unloading of O_2 to tissues. In carbon monoxide poisoning, the curve is shifted to the left and plateaus. (B) Blood gas exchange in tissues and lung alveoli. In tissues, carbon dioxide is generated and freely diffuses into RBCs. In RBCs, carbon dioxide combines with water to form hydrogen ions (H^+) and bicarbonate (HCO_3^-) in a reaction catalyzed by **carbonic anhydrase** (CA). Bicarbonate leaves the RBC in exchange for chloride ion (called the chloride shift) using **band III protein** (*solid black dot*). Carbon dioxide is transported to the lung as bicarbonate in the plasma. The PO_2 within tissues is 40 mm Hg and favors oxygen dissociation from oxyHb to form deoxyHb. The oxygen freely diffuses to tissues. The H^+ is buffered by combining with deoxyHb to form deoxyHb·H^+. In the lung, bicarbonate enters the RBC and combines with H^+ from deoxyHb·H^+ to form carbon dioxide and water in a reaction catalyzed by CA. Carbon dioxide diffuses to lung alveoli and is exhaled. The PO_2 within lung alveoli is 100 mm Hg and favors saturation of deoxyHb with oxygen to form oxyHb.

3. The rate-limiting step in the utilization of oxygen by a cell is the **adenosine diphosphate (ADP) level.**

B. **Clinical considerations**

1. **High-altitude living.** The adaptation to chronic hypoxemia is due in part to **increased synthesis of 2,3-BPG.** When 2,3-BPG binds Hb, the oxygen affinity of Hb is lowered, thereby facilitating unloading of oxygen to tissues. This shifts the Hb–O_2 dissociation curve to the **right.**

2. **Carbon monoxide (CO) poisoning.** CO competes for oxygen-binding sites on Hb because Hb has a higher affinity for CO than for oxygen. This shifts the Hb–O_2 dissociation curve to the **left** and **plateaus** the curve below saturation.

V. WHITE BLOOD CELLS (WBCs or leukocytes)

A. Neutrophils

1. Neutrophils are the most abundant leukocyte in the peripheral circulation (40%–75%).

2. They have a multilobed nucleus.

3. They have primary (azurophilic) granules, which are lysosomes that contain **acid hydrolases** and **myeloperoxidase** (produces hypochlorite ions).

4. Neutrophils have secondary granules that contain **lysozyme, lactoferrin, alkaline phosphatase,** and other **bacteriostatic and bacteriocidal substances.**

5. They have **respiratory burst oxidase** (a membrane enzyme), which produces hydrogen peroxide and superoxide, which kill bacteria.

6. Neutrophils are the first to arrive at an area of tissue damage (within 30 minutes; **acute inflammation**), being attracted to the site by complement C5a and leukotriene B_4.

7. They are highly adapted for **anaerobic glycolysis** with large amounts of glycogen to function in a devascularized area.

8. Neutrophils play an important role in **phagocytosis of bacteria and dead cells** by using **antibody receptors (Fc portion), complement factors,** and **bacterial polysaccharides** to bind to the foreign material. Neutrophils must bind to the foreign material to begin phagocytosis.

9. They impart **natural (or innate) immunity** along with macrophages and natural killer (NK) cells.

B. Eosinophils

1. Eosinophils comprise **5%** of the leukocytes in the peripheral circulation.

2. They have a bi-lobed nucleus.

3. They have highly eosinophilic granules that contain **major basic protein, acid hydrolases,** and **peroxidase.**

4. Eosinophils have **immunoglobulin E (IgE) antibody receptors.**

5. They play a role in **parasitic infection** (e.g., schistosomiasis, ascariasis, trichinosis).

6. They play a role in **reducing the severity of allergic reactions** by secreting histaminase and prostaglandins E1 and E2, which degrade histamine (secreted by mast cells) and inhibit mast cell secretion, respectively.

C. Basophils

1. Basophils comprise 0.5% of the leukocytes in the peripheral circulation (i.e., the least abundant leukocyte).

2. They have highly basophilic granules that contain **heparin, histamine, 5-hydroxytryptamine,** and **sulfated proteoglycans.**

3. They have **IgE antibody receptors.**

4. Basophils play a role in immediate (type I) hypersensitivity reactions (anaphylactic reactions) causing **allergic rhinitis (hay fever), some forms of asthma, urticaria,** and **anaphylaxis.**

D. Monocytes

1. Monocytes comprise 1%–5% of the leukocytes in the peripheral circulation.

2. They are members of the **monocyte–macrophage system,** which includes Kupffer cells in liver, alveolar macrophages, histiocytes in connective tissue, microglia in brain, Langerhans cells in skin, osteoclasts in bone, and dendritic antigen-presenting cells.

3. Monocytes have granules that are lysosomes that contain **acid hydrolases, aryl sulfatase, acid phosphatase,** and **peroxidase.**

4. They respond to dead cells, microorganisms, and inflammation by leaving the peripheral circulation to enter tissues and are then called macrophages.

5. Monocytes impart natural (innate) immunity along with neutrophils and NK cells.

E. B lymphocytes and plasma cells

1. **Development before exposure to antigen**
   a. During fetal development, B-cell differentiation occurs in the **bone marrow.**
   b. **Pro-B cells** and **pre-B cells** undergo heavy-chain gene rearrangement.
   c. **Immature B** cells begin light-chain rearrangement and express antigen-specific IgM on the cell surface.
   d. **Mature (or virgin) B cells** express **antigen-specific IgM and IgD** on the cell surface.
   e. Mature B cells migrate to spleen, lymph node, and gut-associated tissue and lie in wait for antigen exposure.

2. **Development after exposure to antigen**
   a. **Mature B cells** bind antigen using IgM and IgD. As a consequence, **CD79a** and **CD79b** function as signal transducers and cause proliferation and differentiation of B cells into **plasma cells that secrete IgM or IgD.**
   b. Later in the immune response, mature B cells internalize the antigen–IgM or antigen–IgD complex, and the complex undergoes degradation in **endosomal acid vesicles.**
   c. Some of the antigen peptide fragments become associated with **class II major histocompatibility complex (MHC)** and are exposed on the cell surface of the mature B cell.
   d. The antigen peptide–class II MHC is recognized by **CD4+ helper T cells,** which secrete **interleukin-2 (IL-2).**
   e. Under the influence of CD4+ helper T cells and IL-2, mature B cells undergo **isotype switching,** which allows B cells to differentiate into plasma cells that secrete IgG, IgE, or IgA, and **hypermutation,** which produces antibodies that bind with greater affinity.

3. B cells, plasma cells, and immunoglobulins are the basis of **humoral response.**

4. B memory cells are programmed to react to the same antigen upon re-exposure to that antigen, resulting in a faster immune response called the **secondary immune response.** The immunoglobulin secreted by B memory cells has a higher affinity for the antigen that the immunoglobulin produced during the initial exposure due to hypermutation. This is the basis of **immunization.**

F. T lymphocytes

    1. Development before exposure to antigen
      a. In fetal development, T-cell differentiation occurs in the **thymus.**
      b. Pre-T cells begin T-cell receptor (TcR) gene rearrangement.
      c. Immature T cells express antigen-specific TcR, CD4, and CD8 on the cell surface.
      d. Immature T cells undergo the following processes:
        (1) Positive selection, whereby only those T cells that bind with a certain affinity to MHC proteins on thymic epitheliocytes survive (all other T cells undergo apoptosis)
        (2) Negative selection, whereby T cells that recognized "self" antigens undergo apoptosis, leaving T cells that recognize only foreign antigens
      e. Mature T cells downregulate either CD4 or CD8 and leave the thymus. Mature T cells are never both CD4+ and CD8+.
      f. Mature T cells migrate to the **thymic-dependent zone of lymph nodes** and to the **periarterial lymphatic sheath in the spleen,** where they lie in wait for antigen exposure.

    2. Development after exposure to antigen
      a. Exogenous antigens circulating in the bloodstream are phagocytosed by antigen-presenting cells and undergo degradation in endosomal acid vesicles. Antigen proteins are degraded into antigen peptide fragments, which are presented on the cell surface in conjunction with class II MHC. **CD4+ helper T cells** with antigen-specific TcR on their cell surfaces recognize the antigen peptide fragment.
      b. Endogenous antigens (virus or bacteria with a cell) are processed within the rough endoplasmic reticulum into antigen peptide fragments, which are presented on the cell surface in conjunction with class I MHC. **CD8+ cytotoxic T cells** with antigen-specific TcR on its cell surface recognize the antigen peptide fragment.

    3. CD4+ helper T cells promote B-cell differentiation and are depleted in patients with AIDS.

    4. CD8+ cytotoxic T cells are the basis of **cell-mediated immune response.**

    5. Suppressor T cells are either CD4+ or CD8+ and **inhibit** the activity of cytotoxic T cells and helper T cells.

    6. Memory T cells are programmed to react to the same antigen upon re-exposure to that antigen, resulting in a faster cell-mediated immune response.

G. NK cells play an important role in the elimination of virus-infected cells and tumor cells not previously encountered. They impart natural (innate) immunity along with neutrophils and macrophages.

VI. HYPERSENSITIVITY REACTIONS. In addition to providing protection, the immune system may produce deleterious reactions called **hypersensitivity** or **allergic reactions,** which include the following:

A. **Type I anaphylactic reactions** are mediated by IgE (i.e., **antibody-mediated**), which binds to antibody receptors on basophils and mast cells. When cross-linked by antigens, IgE triggers basophils and mast cells to release their contents. Reaction occurs within **minutes.** Clinically, this type of reaction occurs in a wide spectrum ranging from **rashes** and **wheal-and-flare reactions** to **anaphylactic shock.**

B. **Type II cytotoxic reactions** are mediated by IgG or IgM (i.e., **antibody-mediated**), which bind to antigen on the surface of a cell and kill the cell through complement activation. Clinically, this type of reaction occurs in **blood transfusion reactions, Rh incompatibility, transplant rejection via antibodies, drug-induced thrombocytopenia purpura, hemolytic anemia,** and **autoimmune diseases.**

C. **Type III immune complex reactions** are mediated by **antigen–antibody complexes** (i.e., **antibody-mediated**) that activate complement, which in turn activates neutrophils and macrophages to cause tissue damage. Reaction occurs within **hours.** Clinically, this type of reaction occurs in **serum sickness, chronic glomerulonephritis, poststreptococcal glomerulonephritis, rheumatoid arthritis, systemic lupus erythematosus, polyarteritis nodosa, Farmer's lung,** and the **Arthus reaction.**

D. **Type IV delayed-type reactions** are mediated by **T cells** (i.e., **cell-mediated**). This type of reaction takes longer to mount (**1–2 days**) than antibody-mediated reactions (types I–III) due to the time it takes to mobilize T cells through a cascade of activation events. Clinically, this type of reaction occurs in **poison ivy dermatitis (contact sensitivity),** whereby Langerhans cells (antigen-presenting cells) in the skin respond to **urushiol** (an oil); **transplant rejection via cells; tuberculin reaction (Mycobacterium tuberculosis; purified protein derivative skin test); sarcoidosis; Crohn's disease;** and **ulcerative colitis.**

VII. PLATELETS

A. Characteristics

1. Platelets are cell fragments derived from **megakaryocytes.**

2. They are involved in **hemostasis (blood clotting).**

3. They have α-granules that contain **platelet factor 4, platelet-derived growth factor (PDGF), factor V,** and **fibrinogen.**

4. They have δ-granules that contain **serotonin, ADP,** and **calcium.**

B. Clinical considerations

1. Platelet activation by either collagen or thrombin causes release of **arachidonic acid** from the cell membrane, which is converted to **thromboxane A_2.** Thromboxane A_2 stimulates platelet secretion.

2. A severe reduction in the number of circulating platelets is called **thrombocytopenia,** which causes spontaneous bleeding and manifests in skin as small reddish-purple blotches called **purpura.**

VIII. HEMOSTASIS (Figure 9-2)

A. Two pathways

1. Extrinsic pathway
   a. Damaged tissue releases **thromboplastin.**
   b. Thromboplastin initiates a cascade involving **factors VII, X, V,** and **prothrombin activator.**
   c. Prothrombin activator converts **prothrombin to thrombin.**

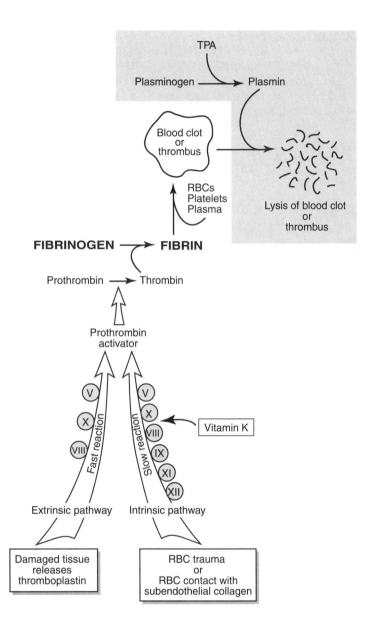

Figure 9-2.   Diagram of hemostasis. The extrinsic and intrinsic pathways are depicted, both of which lead to the production of prothrombin activator. Prothrombin activator converts prothrombin to thrombin. Thrombin subsequently converts fibrinogen to fibrin. Vitamin K is essential for hemostasis. The *shaded box* indicates the mechanism for lysis of the blood clot or thrombus. Tissue plasminogen activator (*TPA*) converts plasminogen to plasmin. Plasmin initiates lysis.

     d. Thrombin converts **fibrinogen to fibrin.**

     e. Fibrin, along with RBCs, platelets, and plasma, forms a **blood clot,** or **thrombus.**

  2. Intrinsic pathway

     a. RBC trauma or RBC contact with subendothelial collagen initiates a cascade involving **factors XII, XI, IX, VIII, X, V, and prothrombin activator.**

     b. Prothrombin activator converts **prothrombin to thrombin.**

     c. Thrombin converts **fibrinogen to fibrin.**

     d. Fibrin, along with RBCs, platelets, and plasma, forms a **blood clot,** or **thrombus.**

B. **Vitamin K** is essential for hemostasis because it acts as a cofactor for an enzyme that forms **γ-carboxyglutamate residues** in certain blood factor proteins. This allows factor proteins to bind to cell membranes because γ-carboxyglutamate residues have a high affinity for **calcium.**

  1. **Vitamin K deficiency** can result in hemorrhage. However, adult vitamin K deficiency is rare because intestinal bacteria produce 50% of the required vitamin K.

  2. **Dicumarol** and **warfarin** are vitamin K analogues that inhibit hemostasis.

C. Hemophilia

  1. In patients with **hemophilia A** (the most common type of hemophilia), **factor VIII** is absent.

  2. In patients with **hemophilia B, factor IX** is absent.

IX. SELECTED PHOTOMICROGRAPHS

  A. Hereditary spherocytosis, β-thalassemia major, sickle cell disease, and G6PD deficiency (Figure 9-3)

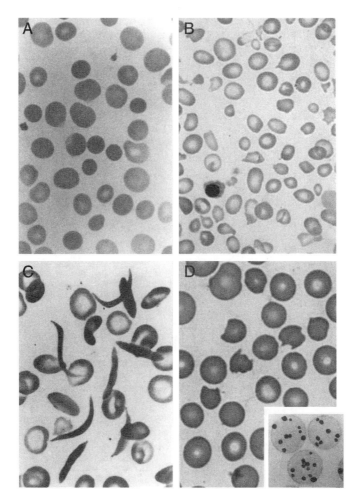

Figure 9-3. (A) Hereditary spherocytosis, a genetic disease characterized by a deficiency in the spectrin protein that helps stabilize the RBC membrane, usually is caused by a mutation of the ankyrin gene. This results in aniso-cytosis (variation in size of RBCs) and spherocytes with no central pallor zone. The osmotic fragility test is the con-firmatory test for hereditary spherocytosis. (Reprinted with permission from Stiene-Martin EA, Lotspeich-Steininger CA, Koepke JA: *Clinical Hematology,* 2nd ed. Philadelphia, Lippincott, 1998, p 91.) (B) β-thalassemia major is shown with some large, polychromatic RBCs that are newly released from the bone marrow in response to the anemia. However, most RBCs are small (microcytic) and colorless (hypochromic). Also apparent are many ir-regular-shaped RBCs (poikilocytes) that have been traumatized or damaged during passage through the spleen. (Courtesy of Jean Shafer; Department of Medicine; University of Rochester from web site jrutherford@cjp.com, Carden Jennings Publishing Co. Ltd.) (C) Sickle cell anemia is shown with sickle RBCs (depranocytes) due to the rod-shaped polymers of the inherited abnormal hemoglobin S (HbS). The RBC does not become sickled until it has lost its nucleus and has its full complement of HbS. Sickle cells are thin, elongated, and well-filled with HbS. The main clinical manifestations of sickle cell disease are chronic hemolytic anemia and occlusion of microvascu-lature (called vaso-occlusive disease). Vaso-occlusive crisis may occur in the brain, liver, lung, or spleen. Factors that induce sickling are PO_2 (e.g., high altitude) or a concentration of 60% HbS or greater in RBCs. (Reprinted with permission from Stiene-Martin EA, Lotspeich-Steininger CA, Koepke JA: *Clinical Hematology,* 2nd ed. Philadelphia, Lippincott, 1998, p 96.) (D) Glucose-6-phosphate dehydrogenase (G6PD) deficiency is a genetic dis-ease in which the deficiency reduces the ability of RBCs to protect themselves from oxidative injury. This leads to a denaturation of Hb, which forms Hb precipitates within the RBC (*see inset*) called Heinz bodies. As these RBCs percolate through the spleen, splenic macrophages "chew" the Heinz bodies so that RBCs have a "bite" of cyto-plasm removed and are called *bite cells*. However, the majority of RBCs are normocytic and normochromatic. (Courtesy of Jean Shafer; Department of Medicine; University of Rochester from web site jrutherford@cjp.com, Carden Jennings Publishing Co. Ltd. Inset reprinted with permission from Stiene-Martin EA, Lotspeich-Steininger CA, Koepke JA: *Clinical Hematology,* 2nd ed. Philadelphia, Lippincott, 1998, p 99.)

B. Vitamin B$_{12}$ deficiency, lead poisoning, iron deficiency, Howell-Jolly bodies (Figure 9-4)

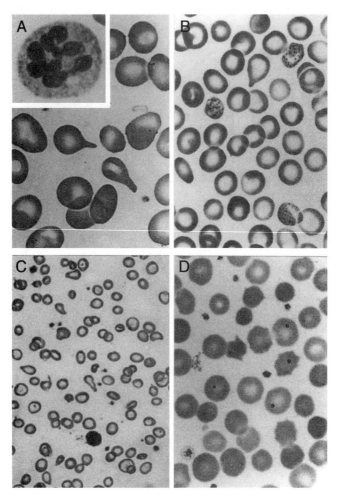

Figure 9-4.   (A) Pernicious anemia due to vitamin B$_{12}$ deficiency caused by atrophic gastritis with decreased intrinsic factor production. Some RBCs are deformed as they pass through the splenic sinuses and appear teardrop shaped (dacryocytes). In addition, large neutrophils with a hypersegmented nucleus (five to six lobes) can be observed (*inset*). (Reprinted with permission from Stiene-Martin EA, Lotspeich-Steininger CA, Koepke JA: *Clinical Hematology*, 2nd ed. Philadelphia, Lippincott, 1998, p 95. Inset reprinted with permission from Carr JH, Rodak BF: *Clinical Hematology Atlas*. Philadelphia, Saunders, 1999, p 143.) (B) Lead poisoning is shown in which the RBCs are microcytic, are hypochromic, and show basophilic stippling, which probably represents breakdown of ribosomes. Lead denatures sulfhydryl (SH) groups in ferrochelatase within mitochondria that bind iron to protoporphyrin to form heme, thus inhibiting hemoglobin synthesis. As a result, unbound iron accumulates in mitochondria and forms ringed sideroblasts. (Reprinted with permission from Stiene-Martin EA, Lotspeich-Steininger CA, Koepke JA: *Clinical Hematology*, 2nd ed. Philadelphia, Lippincott, 1998, p 98.) (C) Iron deficiency anemia is shown with RBCs that are microcytic and hypochromic with a thin rim of Hb at the periphery. Iron deficiency is probably the most common nutritional disorder in the world. Iron is stored in the body as ferritin within the cytoplasm of cells and as hemosiderin within lysosomes. Some ferritin normally circulates in the plasma and is a good indicator of iron stores (iron deficiency: < 12 µg/l; iron overload: 5000 µg/l). Iron is transported in the body mainly by transferrin, which is synthesized by the liver. The main function of transferrin is to deliver iron to cells, particularly to RBC precursors, which need iron for Hb synthesis. (Courtesy of Jean Shafer; Department of Medicine; University of Rochester from web site jrutherford@cjp.com, Carden Jennings Publishing Co. Ltd.) (D) Howell-Jolly bodies after splenectomy. Howell-Jolly bodies represent nuclear fragments that are normally removed from RBCs as they pass through the splenic sinuses. After splenectomy, increased numbers of RBCs with these inclusions are observed. (Reprinted with permission from Stiene-Martin EA, Lotspeich-Steininger CA, Koepke JA: *Clinical Hematology*, 2nd ed. Philadelphia, Lippincott, 1998, p 97.)

C. Spur cells in alcoholic cirrhosis, burr cells in kidney failure, target cells (Figure 9-5)

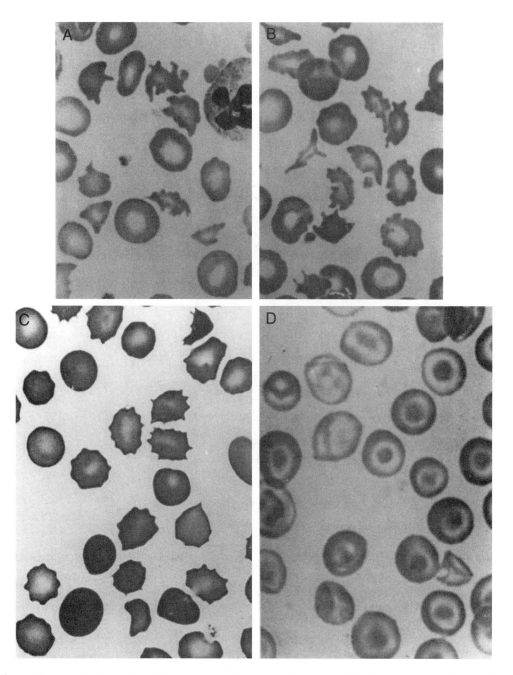

Figure 9-5.   (*A and B*) Hemolytic anemia associated with alcoholic cirrhosis shows RBCs with a periphery consisting of sharp points called *spur cells*. (C) Anemia associated with kidney failure (or renal insufficiency) shows RBCs with a periphery consisting of bumps called *burr cells*. (D) *Target cells* (or codocytes) have a central dark area of Hb that is surrounded by a colorless ring followed by a peripheral rim of Hb. Target cells can be found in a number of pathologic states, including thalassemia, obstructive liver disease, and iron deficiency. (Reprinted with permission from Stiene-Martin EA, Lotspeich-Steininger CA, Koepke JA: *Clinical Hematology*, 2nd ed. Philadelphia, Lippincott, 1998, pp 92–93).

D. Chronic myeloid leukemia (Figure 9-6)

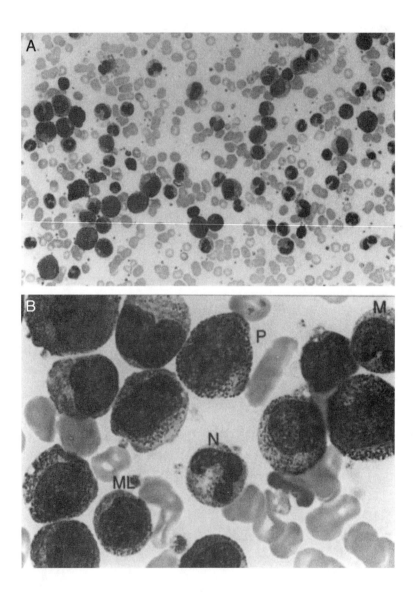

Figure 9-6. Chronic myeloid leukemia (CML). (A) Low-power light micrograph showing an increased number of granulocytes in all stages of maturation and many mature neutrophils. (B) Higher-power light micrograph showing neutrophils (*N*), metamyelocytes (*M*), myelocytes (*ML*), and promyelocytes (*P*). A characteristic finding in CML is the absence of alkaline phosphatase in granulocytes. The absence of alkaline phosphatase activity is used to distinguish CML from a leukemoid reaction. In 90% of CML cases, the **Philadelphia (Ph) chromosome,** which is a reciprocal translocation of DNA involving band q34 on chromosome 9 and band q11 on chromosome 22 [t(9;22)(q34;q11)], is found. This translocation results in the *bcr-c-abl* fusion gene, which codes for a protein with tyrosine kinase activity. (Reprinted with permission from Mufti GJ, Flandrin G, Schaefer H-E, et al: *An Atlas of Malignant Haematology.* Philadelphia, Lippincott-Raven, 1996, p 179.)

E. Chronic lymphocytic leukemia (Figure 9-7)

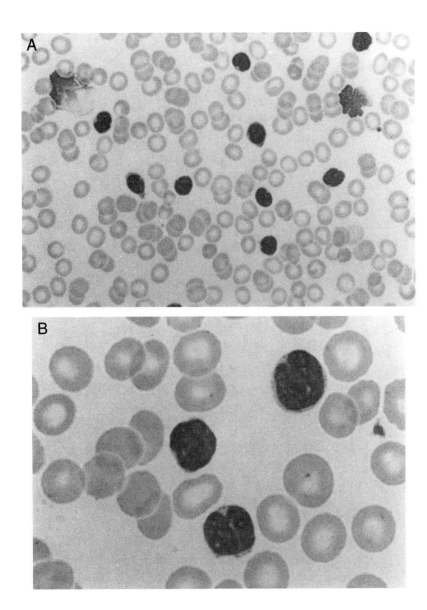

Figure 9-7.   Chronic lymphocytic leukemia (CLL). (A) Low-power light micrograph showing an increased number of small, mature-looking B lymphocytes. (B) Higher-power light micrograph showing B lymphocytes with condensed nuclear chromatin and a high nucleus:cytoplasm ratio. CLL, which is the most common leukemia, is a disorder of mature (virgin) B cells that are unable to differentiate into plasma cells, causing hypogammaglobulinemia. (Reprinted with permission from Mufti GJ, Flandrin G, Schaefer H-E, et al: *An Atlas of Malignant Haematology*. Philadelphia, Lippincott-Raven, 1996, p 225.)

F. Hairy cell leukemia, Reed-Sternberg cells, Chediak-Higashi syndrome (Figure 9-8)

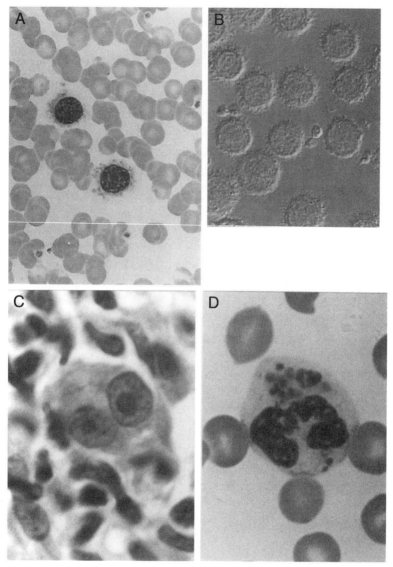

Figure 9-8.   (*A and B*) Hairy cell leukemia. (A) B lymphocytes are shown with prominent cytoplasmic projections. (Reprinted with permission from Mufti GJ, Flandrin G, Schaefer H-E, et al: *An Atlas of Malignant Haematology*. Philadelphia, Lippincott-Raven, 1996, p 244.) (B) Nomarski interference illumination clearly showing B lymphocytes with prominent cytoplasmic projections. Hairy cell leukemia is a relatively rare but distinctive form of chronic B lymphocyte leukemia that receives its name because of the distinctive feature of the cytoplasmic projections of the B lymphocyte. Massive splenomegaly is the most common physical finding. A positive tartrate-resistant acid phosphatase stain is a key to confirming the diagnosis. (Reprinted with permission from Mufti GJ, Flandrin G, Schaefer H-E, et al: *An Atlas of Malignant Haematology*. Philadelphia, Lippincott-Raven, 1996, p 242.) (C) A Reed-Sternberg cell is a distinctive giant cell that is considered an essential neoplastic element in Hodgkin disease. The Reed-Sternberg cell is often binucleate or bilobed with a prominent nucleolus. (Reprinted with permission from Gatter K, Brown D: *An Illustrated Guide to Bone Marrow Diagnosis*. Malden, MA, Blackwell Science, 1997, p 134.) (*D*) Chediak-Higashi syndrome is a genetic disease characterized by neutropenia and impaired phagocytosis of bacteria due to a defect in microtubule polymerization. Large abnormal lysosomes can be observed in the cytoplasm of a neutrophil. (Reprinted with permission from Carr JH, Rodak BF: *Clinical Hematology Atlas*. Philadelphia, Saunders, 1999, p 143.)

G. Neutrophil (Figure 9-9; see V A)

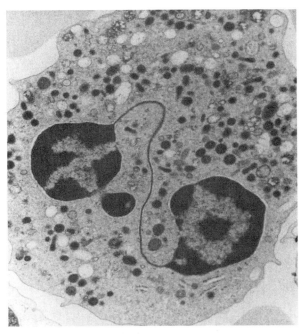

Figure 9-9.   Electron micrograph of a neutrophil. Although neutrophilic granules show considerable hetero-
geneity, two types are described: *primary* (azurophilic) granules, which are lysosomes, and *secondary* granules.
Note the multilobed nucleus. (Courtesy of J. Parkin, University of Minnesota, Minneapolis, Minnesota)

H. Eosinophil (Figure 9-10; see V B)

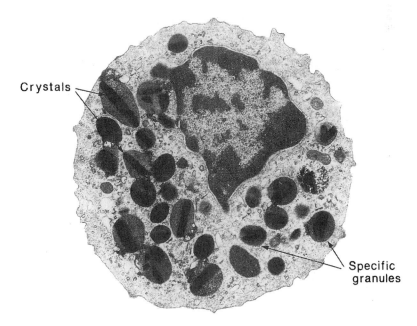

Crystals

Specific
granules

Figure 9-10.   Electron micrograph of an eosinophil. Note the conspicuous crystals within the granules. Although not apparent in this electron micrograph, the nucleus is bi-lobed. (Reprinted with permission from Fawcett
DW: A *Textbook of Histology*, 12th ed. New York, Chapman Hall, 1994, p 197. Courtesy of Don W. Fawcett, M.D.)

I. Lymphocyte, plasma cell (Figure 9-11; see V E)

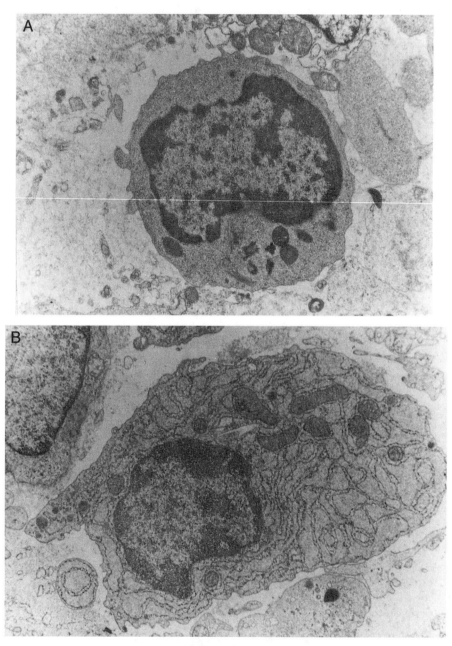

Figure 9-11. (A) Electron micrograph of a lymphocyte . (Courtesy of J. Parkin, University of Minnesota, Minneapolis, Minnesota). (B) Electron micrograph of a plasma cell. Although plasma cells secrete immunoglobulins (proteins), secretory granules are not observed. These cells possess a prominent Golgi complex, known as the Hof area (not clearly shown), and extensive rough endoplasmic reticulum (rER). Lymphocytes and plasma cells are related because B lymphocytes differentiate into plasma cells. (Reprinted with permission from Erlandsen SL, Magney JE: *Human Histology: A Microfiche Atlas*. Minneapolis, University of Minnesota Press, 1985.)

10
Thymus

I. THYMIC CORTEX (Figure 10-1) consists of:

A. Immature T cells (also called thymocytes)

B. Thymic epitheliocytes

1. Thymic epitheliocytes form a cellular meshwork into which immature T cells are tightly packed.
2. They secrete **thymosin, serum thymic factor,** and **thymopoietin,** which transform immature T cells into mature T cells.
3. They secrete **thymotaxin,** which attracts progenitor T cells (stem cells) from the bone marrow to populate the thymus.
4. Thymic epitheliocytes are derived embryologically from **endoderm.**
5. They are joined by **desmosomes** and contain **cytokeratin** intermediate filaments.
6. They are sometimes called **thymic nurse cells.**

II. THYMIC MEDULLA consists of the following:

A. Mature T cells

B. Thymic epitheliocytes

C. Thymic (Hassall's) corpuscles, which are whorl-like structures composed of keratinized thymic epitheliocytes (see Figure 10-1)

III. MATURATION OF T CELLS (see Chapter 9 V E). As T cells mature, they express:

A. T-cell receptors (TcR) that are antigen-specific

B. Cluster of differentiation (CD) surface markers

1. Helper T cells are CD4+.
2. Cytotoxic T cells are CD8+.
3. Suppressor T cells are either CD4+ or CD8+.

IV. BLOOD–THYMUS BARRIER

A. The blood–thymus barrier is found only in the thymic cortex.

B. This barrier assures that immature T cells undergo maturation in an antigen-free environment.

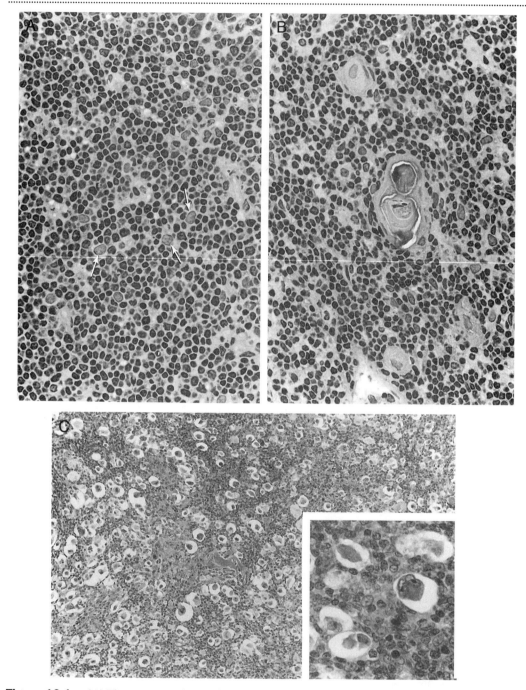

Figure 10-1.   (A) Thymic cortex shows a large number of densely packed immature T cells of various sizes. In addition , thymic epitheliocytes (*arrows*) are apparent. (B) Thymic medulla showing the whorl-like Hassall's corpuscles, which are keratinized thymic epitheliocytes. (C) Thymoma is a tumor of thymic epitheliocytes. A huge proliferation of thymic epitheliocytes occurs (compare with normal thymus in A). *Inset* shows high magnification of thymic epitheliocytes. Note that this figure shows thymic epitheliocytes in three different states: normal (in A), keratinized (in B), and tumorous (in C). (C: Reprinted with permission from the East Carolina University, School of Medicine, Department of Pathology slide collection.)

C. It consists of tight junctions between nonfenestrated endothelial cells, basal lamina, and thymic epitheliocytes.

V. INVOLUTION OF THE THYMUS

A. At birth, the thymus is fully developed.

B. In early childhood, involution begins.

C. At puberty, involution greatly accelerates.

D. By early adulthood, the thymus is transformed primarily into adipose tissue with isolated areas of lymphatic tissue.

    1. Despite the apparent involution, the thymus remains a source of T cells throughout life.

    2. Involution can be accelerated by stress, adrenocorticotrophic hormone (ACTH), or steroids.

VI. THYMECTOMY

A. **Neonatal thymectomy** severely impairs cell-mediated immunity and also somewhat diminishes humoral immunity because helper T-cell function is compromised. The lymph nodes and spleen are reduced in size because the thymic-dependent zone of the lymph nodes and periarterial lymphatic sheath of the spleen, respectively, do not become populated with T cells.

B. **Adult thymectomy** causes less severe impairment of cell-mediated immunity and humoral immunity because the lymph nodes and spleen are already well populated with long-lived T cells.

11
Lymph Node

I. OUTER CORTEX consists of the following:

   A. B cells (see Chapter 9 V E), which are organized into **lymphatic follicles** that may contain germinal centers (these are evidence of an immune response whereby B cells are transformed into plasma cells)

   B. Helper T cells

   C. Follicular dendritic cells, which have an antigen-presenting function

   D. Macrophages

   E. Fibroblasts (reticular cells), which secrete type III collagen (reticular fibers) that form a stromal meshwork

II. INNER CORTEX (paracortex; thymic-dependent zone) consists of the following:

   A. T cells

   B. Dendritic cells, which have an antigen-presenting function

   C. Macrophages

   D. Fibroblasts (reticular cells), which secrete type III collagen (reticular fibers) that form a stromal meshwork

III. MEDULLA consists of the following:

   A. Lymphocytes

   B. Plasma cells

   C. Macrophages, which are very numerous in the medulla (therefore, phagocytosis is extremely active)

   D. Fibroblasts (reticular cells), which secrete type III collagen (reticular fibers) that form a stromal meshwork

IV. FLOW OF LYMPH occurs through afferent lymphatics, subcapsular (marginal) sinus, cortical sinuses, medullary sinuses, and finally through efferent lymphatics. Sinuses contain sinus macrophages, veiled cells, and reticular fibers that crisscross the lumen in a haphazard fashion.

V. FLOW OF BLOOD occurs through arteries that enter at the hilum, a capillary network within the outer and inner cortex, postcapillary (high endothelial) venules within the inner cortex, and veins that leave at the hilum. Postcapillary (high endothelial) venules

have **lymphocyte homing receptors** and are the site where lymphocytes exit the bloodstream to repopulate the lymph node.

VI. CLINICAL CONSIDERATION (Figure 11-1). The population of lymphocytes within lymph nodes changes in certain clinical states, such as agammaglobulinemia, DiGeorge syndrome, and severe combined immunodeficiency (SCID) or adenosine deaminase deficiency (ADA; "bubble boy" disease).

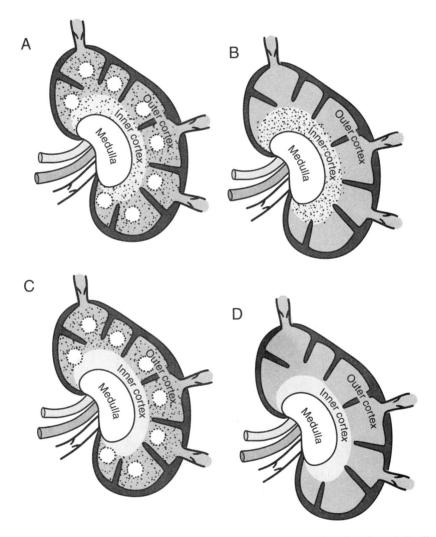

Figure 11-1. Diagram of lymph nodes in various clinical states. (A) Normal lymph node with B cells (outer cortex) and T cells (inner cortex) that impart a humoral immune response and cell-mediated immune response to the individual, respectively. (B) Lymph node in X-linked infantile (Bruton's) agammaglobulinemia with B cells absent but T cells present, so that humoral immune response is absent but cell-mediated immune response is present. (C) Lymph node in DiGeorge syndrome with B cells present but T cells absent, so that humoral immune response is present but cell-mediated immune response is absent. (D) Lymph node in severe combined immunodeficiency disease (SCID) or adenosine deaminase deficiency (ADA; "bubble boy" disease) with B cells and T cells absent, so that both humoral immune response and cell-mediated immune response are absent.

VII. SELECTED PHOTOMICROGRAPHS. Normal lymph node, lymph node in patient with late-stage AIDS, and lymph node in patient with breast cancer metastasis (Figure 11-2).

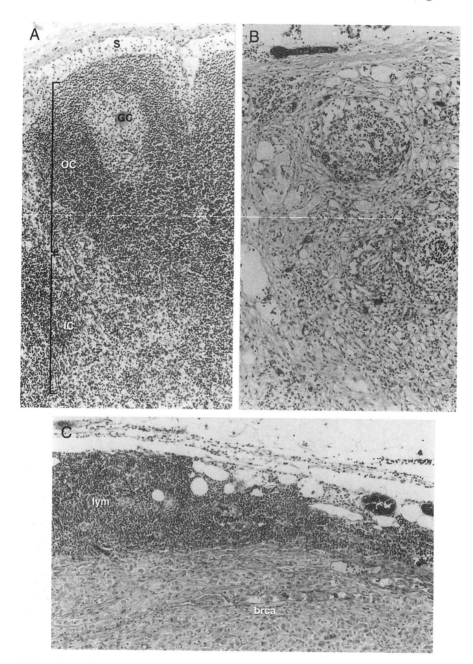

Figure 11-2. (A) Light micrograph of a normal lymph node showing the subcapsular sinus (*s*), outer cortex (OC), inner cortex (IC), and germinal center (GC) of a lymphatic follicle. (B) Lymph node in late-stage AIDS showing a marked reduction in lymphocytes, especially in the inner cortex. (C) Lymph node with breast cancer metastasis showing lymphoid tissue (*lym*) crowded to the periphery by the invasion of breast cancer cells (*brca*). (B, C: Reprinted with permission from East Carolina University, School of Medicine, Department of Pathology slide collection.)

12

Spleen

I. WHITE PULP (Figure 12-1) consists of the following:

A. B cells, which are organized into **lymphatic follicles** that surround a central artery

B. T cells, which are organized into a sheath around a central artery called the **periarterial lymphatic sheath (PALS),** which is a **thymic-dependent zone** similar to the inner cortex of a lymph node

II. MARGINAL ZONE is located between the white pulp and red pulp. It is the **site of immune response initiation,** which occurs in the spleen as foreign antigens encounter antigen-presenting cells. The marginal zone consists of the following:

A. Macrophages

B. Antigen-presenting cells

III. RED PULP is organized into **splenic (Billroth) cords,** which are separated by splenic sinuses. It is the **site of red blood cell (RBC) removal** [i.e., senescent, damaged, or genetically altered (e.g., sickle cell disease) RBCs] from the circulation by macrophages. The red pulp consists of the following:

A. Macrophages

B. Plasma cells

C. Lymphocytes

D. RBCs

IV. BLOOD FLOW through the spleen involves the splenic artery, trabecular arteries, central arteries, penicillar (straight) arterioles, splenic sinuses, trabecular veins, and the splenic vein.

V. CLINICAL CONSIDERATIONS

A. Howell-Jolly bodies are found after splenectomy and represent nuclear fragments that are normally removed from RBCs as they pass through the splenic sinuses. After splenectomy, increased numbers of RBCs with Howell-Jolly bodies are observed.

B. After splenectomy, the risk of ***Streptococcus pneumoniae*** septicemia increases, so anyone undergoing a splenectomy should be immunized against S. *pneumoniae*. The S. *pneumoniae* bacteria stays primarily in the bloodstream; thus, the lymph nodes do not respond to it well, and the immune response is mounted by the spleen.

C. Congestive splenomegaly is usually due to portal hypertension caused by cirrhosis.

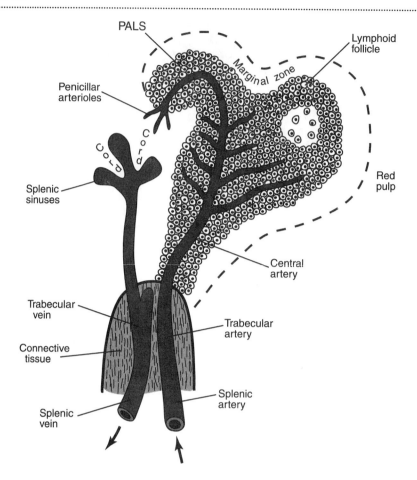

Figure 12-1.   Diagram of normal splenic architecture and vascular pattern. *PALS* = peri-arterial lymphatic sheath. (Modified from Faller DV: Diseases of the spleen. In *Cecil Textbook of Medicine*, 18th ed. Edited by Wyngaarden JB, Smith LH. Philadelphia, Saunders, 1988, p 1036.)

The spleen is frequently covered by a "sugar-coated" capsule and focal areas of fibrosis containing iron and calcium called **Gandy-Gamna nodules.**

D. Felty syndrome is a syndrome with the combined features of rheumatoid arthritis, splenomegaly, and neutropenia.

13
Stomach

I. MUCOSA is lined by **surface mucous cells** that are attached by juxtaluminal tight junctions and that secrete mucus to protect the mucosa from the acid pH and hydrolytic enzymes contained in the gastric juice.

II. GASTRIC GLANDS contain the following cell types:

A. **Stem cells,** which play a role in regeneration

B. **Mucous neck cells**

C. **Parietal cells** (Figure 13-1), which secrete the following:

    1. **Hydrochloric acid (HCl)** is secreted into the gastric lumen. HCl is produced through the action of **carbonic anhydrase** and **H^+–K^+–adenosine triphosphatase (ATPase)** (a H^+ pump). Cl^- are secreted along with H^+, so the secretion product of parietal cells is HCl.

    2. **Bicarbonate (HCO_3^-)** secreted into the bloodstream causes an increase in the pH called the **alkaline tide.**

    3. **Intrinsic factor** is necessary for **vitamin B_{12} absorption. Pernicious anemia** may result due to vitamin B_{12} deficiency caused by atrophic gastritis with decreased intrinsic factor production (see Chapter 9; Figure 9-4).

D. **Chief cells** secrete **pepsinogen** (inactive), which is converted to **pepsin** (active) upon contact with the acid pH of the gastric juice.

E. **Enteroendocrine cells**

    1. G cells
        a. These are stimulated **in response to a meal.**
        b. They secrete **gastrin,** which stimulates HCl secretion from parietal cells.
        c. They are found predominately in the antrum of the stomach.
        d. If ulcers occur, the antrum may be resected to reduce the amount of HCl secretion.

    2. EC cells secrete **serotonin,** which increases gut motility.

    3. D cells secrete **somatostatin,** which inhibits secretion of nearby enteroendocrine cells.

    4. A cells secrete **glucagon,** which stimulates hepatic glycogen degradation, thereby increasing blood glucose levels.

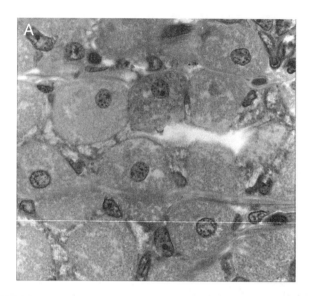

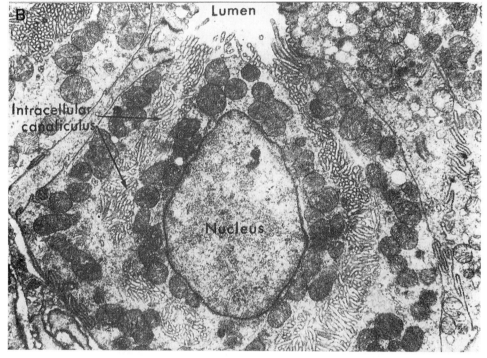

Figure 13-1. (A) Light micrograph of parietal cells. (B) Electron micrograph of a parietal cell. Note the centrally located nucleus, numerous mitochondria, and intracellular canaliculi. (Courtesy of Dr. S. Ito.)

III. GASTRIC EMPTYING describes the process whereby the lower portion of the stomach contracts to move food into the duodenum.

   A. Isotonic stomach contents increase gastric emptying.

   B. Fat inhibits gastric emptying.

   C. H^+ in the duodenal lumen inhibits gastric emptying.

IV. REPAIR (REGENERATION). Stem cells have a high rate of mitosis. They migrate upward to replace surface mucous cells every 4–7 days. Stem cells also may migrate downward to replace mucous neck, parietal, chief, and enteroendocrine cells.

V. CLINICAL CONSIDERATIONS

   A. Gastric ulcers

   1. An ulcer is a breach in the mucosa that extends into the submucosa or deeper.

   2. Ulcers occur where exposure to the aggressive action of the gastric juice is high (e.g., stomach, duodenum, esophagus).

   3. The bacteria *Helicobacter pylori* can contribute to ulcers, so **antibiotics** may be effective in treatment.

   4. **Other treatments** for ulcers include ways to reduce HCl secretion, such as:
   a. **Surgical resection of the pyloric antrum**
   b. **Omeprazole** (an H^+–K^+–ATPase inhibitor)
   c. **Atropine** [a muscarinic ACh receptor (mAChR) antagonist], which blocks the stimulatory effects of ACh released from postganglionic parasympathetic neurons on HCl secretion
   d. **Cimetidine** [a histamine (H_2) receptor antagonist], which blocks the stimulatory effects of histamine released from mast cells on HCl secretion

   B. **Zollinger-Ellison syndrome** is due to a gastrin-secreting tumor of the pancreas that causes increased **H^+ secretion from parietal cells,** which continues unabated because the tumor cells are not subject to feedback inhibition.

14

Small Intestine

I. MUCOSA is lined by the following:

A. Surface absorptive cells

1. These cells are joined by juxtaluminal tight junctions.

2. They possess microvilli that are coated by filamentous glycoproteins called the **glycocalyx.**

    a. The glycocalyx contains the following important enzymes: **lactase, sucrase, maltase, peptidases,** and **enterokinase.**

    b. Enterokinase converts the inactive form (e.g., trypsinogen) of pancreatic enzymes to the active form (e.g., trypsin).

3. Surface absorptive cells absorb carbohydrates, protein, lipids, vitamins, calcium, and iron from the intestinal lumen and transport them to the blood or lymph.

    a. Carbohydrates are digested to monosaccharides (glucose, galactose, fructose). Glucose and galactose are absorbed using a **Na^+-dependent cotransporter.** Fructose is absorbed via facilitated diffusion.

    b. Proteins are digested into amino acids, dipeptides, and tripeptides. These are absorbed using a **Na^+-dependent cotransporter.**

    c. Triacylglycerols (the main fat in a human diet) are emulsified by bile salts and digested to fatty acids and monoacylglycerols.

        (1) Long-chain fatty acids (>12 carbons), monoacylglycerols, cholesterol, and fat-soluble vitamins (A, D, E, and K) are packaged into **micelles** and absorbed.

        (2) Within the surface absorptive cell, **resynthesis of triacylglycerols** occurs in the smooth endoplasmic reticulum (sER). Subsequently, the triacylglycerols, cholesterol, and fat-soluble vitamins are packaged with apoproteins into **chylomicrons** and released into the lymph.

        (3) Short- and medium-chain fatty acids (< 12 carbons) are not packaged into chylomicrons, but are released directly into the portal blood. **Xenical** is a drug used in the treatment of morbid obesity that blocks approximately 30% of dietary fat from being absorbed.

    d. Water-soluble vitamins are absorbed using a **Na^+-dependent cotransporter.** Vitamin B_{12} requires intrinsic factor secreted by parietal cells of the stomach (see Chapter 9, Figure 9-4 and Chapter 13).

    e. Calcium is absorbed and requires 1,25 $(OH)_2$ vitamin D_3, which is produced by the kidney (see Chapter 22), to be fully absorbed.

    f. Iron is absorbed as ferroheme (bound to hemoglobin or myoglobin) or as free Fe^{2+} and transported in the plasma by a protein called **transferrin** (see Chapter 1 VIIIB).

B. **Goblet cells** synthesize **mucinogen,** which is stored in membrane-bound granules.

C. **M cells** are antigen-presenting cells that overlie lymphatic follicles.

II. INTESTINAL GLANDS (CRYPTS OF LIEBERKÜHN) contain the following types of cells:

A. **Stem cells** demonstrate a high rate of mitosis and replace surface absorptive cells and goblet cells every 3–6 days.

B. **Paneth cells** secrete **lysozyme,** which has antibacterial activity (Figure 14-1).

C. **Enteroendocrine cells** (Figure 14-2) are comprised of the following:

1. **I cells** secrete **cholecystokinin (CCK)** in response to small peptides, amino acids, and fatty acids within the gut lumen. CCK stimulates **enzyme secretion** from the pancreas and **release of bile** from the gallbladder.

2. **S cells** secrete **secretin** in response to hydrogen ions and fatty acids within the gut lumen. Secretin stimulates the **release of bicarbonate** from the pancreas and from the biliary tract.

3. **K cells** secrete **gastric-inhibitory peptide (GIP)** in response to orally administered glucose, amino acids, and fatty acids in the gut lumen. GIP stimulates **insulin secretion** from pancreatic islets. This explains why an oral glucose load produces higher serum insulin levels than an intravenous glucose load.

4. **L cells** secrete **glucagon-like peptide–1 (GLP-1)** in response to orally administered glucose, amino acids, and fatty acids in the gut lumen.
   a. GLP-1 **stimulates insulin secretion** from pancreatic islets.
   b. GLP-1 **inhibits glucagon secretion** from pancreatic islets.
   c. GLP-1 may be an effective therapeutic agent for patients with **type 2 diabetes** because the stimulatory effect of GLP-1 on insulin secretion is preserved in these patients.

III. GUT-ASSOCIATED LYMPHATIC TISSUE (GALT)

A. **M cells** sample the intestinal contents and present a specific antigen to immature lymphocytes.

B. **Mature lymphocytes** differentiate into plasma cells that secrete specific immunoglobulin A (IgA) antibodies into the lamina propria.

C. The majority of **IgA** within the lamina propria enters the bloodstream and reaches the liver sinusoids.

D. IgA within the **liver sinusoids** binds to receptors on hepatocytes and is endocytosed. At the bile canaliculi, IgA is released into the biliary tract in combination with a portion of its receptor **(secretory piece)** and is known as secretory IgA.

E. **Secretory IgA** enters the intestinal lumen with the bile.

IV. REPAIR (REGENERATION) involves stem cells (see II A).

V. CLINICAL CONSIDERATIONS

A. **Celiac disease** is a hypersensitivity to **gluten** and **gliadin** protein found in wheat and other grains.

1. Upon ingestion of gluten-containing foods, a large number of lymphocytes, plasma

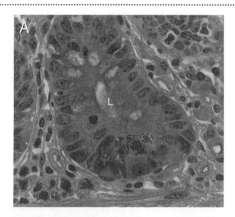

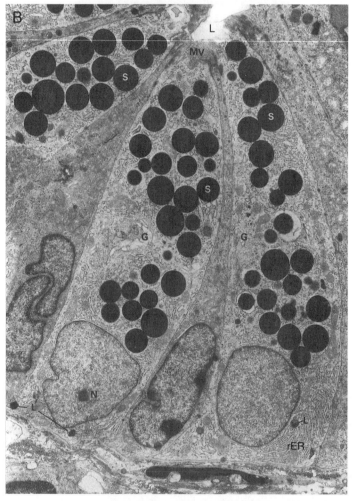

Figure 14-1. (A) Light micrograph of numerous Paneth cells at the base of an intestinal gland with conspicu-ous secretory granules oriented toward the lumen (L). (B) Electron micrograph of Paneth cells. Paneth cells secrete a protein called lysozyme, and therefore, contain secretory granules (S), Golgi complexes (G), and rough endo-plasmic reticulum (rER) typically found in protein-secreting cells. L = lysosomes; MV = microvilli; N = nucleus. (Reprinted with permission from Satoh Y, Yamano M, Matsuda M, et al.: Ultrastructure of pancreatic cells in the intestine. *J Electron Microsc Tech* 16 (1):69, 1990. © 1990, John Wiley & Sons, Inc. Reprinted by permission of Wi-ley-Liss, Inc., a division of John Wiley & Sons, Inc.)

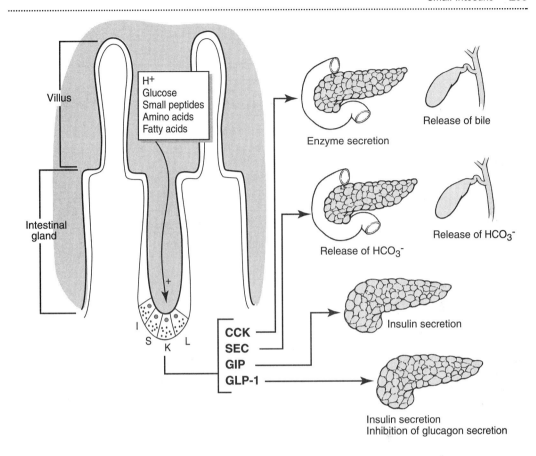

Figure 14-2. Diagram of hormonal secretion from intestinal glands and their actions. Note that hydrogen ions, glucose, small peptides, amino acids, and fatty acids within the lumen of the intestinal gland stimulate the I cells (*I*), S cells (*S*), K cells (*K*), and L cells (*L*). *CCK* = cholecystokinin; *GIP* = gastric inhibitory peptide; *GLP-1* = glucagon-like peptide 1; HCO_3^- = bicarbonate; *SEC* = secretin.

cells, macrophages, and eosinophils accumulate within the lamina propria of the intestinal mucosa.

   a. Gliadin antibodies are generally detectable in the blood.

   b. These factors may contribute to the immunologic damage of the mucosa.

   2. It is characterized clinically by chronic diarrhea, flatulence, weight loss, and fatigue.

B. Crohn disease (CD) is a type of inflammatory bowel disease involving the formation of a granuloma. The etiology of CD is unknown.

   1. A classic feature of CD is the **clear demarcation** between diseased bowel segments located directly next to uninvolved normal bowel.

   2. Neutrophils infiltrate the intestinal glands and ultimately destroy them, leading to **ulcers.** With progression of CD, the ulcers coalesce into long, serpentine ulcers (linear ulcers) oriented along the long axis of the bowel.

   3. CD is characterized clinically by intermittent bouts of diarrhea, weight loss, and weakness.

4. Complications may include strictures of the intestinal lumen and the formation of fistulas.

C. **Cholera** is caused by the gram-negative bacteria ***Vibrio cholerae,*** which produces an enterotoxin called **cholera toxin.**

1. Cholera toxin is an enzyme that catalyzes **adenosine diphosphate (ADP) ribosylation** of the α_S chain of G_S protein. This effectively increases cyclic adenosine monophosphate (cAMP) levels, which activates chloride ion channels of surface absorptive cells to secrete chloride ions into the lumen; sodium ions and water follow.

2. Certain strains of ***Escherichia coli*** produce toxins that cause traveler's diarrhea by a similar mechanism.

3. Both CD and traveler's diarrhea are characterized clinically by a severe, watery diarrhea.

D. **Lactose intolerance** is due to the absence of the enzyme **lactase** from the glycocalyx so that lactose cannot be digested to glucose.

1. The unabsorbed lactose within the lumen results in **osmotic diarrhea.**

2. Congenital lactase deficiency is a rare condition that becomes apparent in infants at the start of milk feeding.

3. Acquired lactase deficiency is generally due to rotavirus gastroenteritis, kwashiorkor, or old age.

4. Is characterized clinically by abdominal distention and an explosive, watery diarrhea.

15

Large Intestine (Colon)

I. ANAL CANAL

A. **The upper anal canal** is separated from the lower anal canal by the **pectinate line** (Figure 15-1).

    1. The upper anal canal is lined by a typical simple columnar (colonic) epithelium arranged as intestinal glands (Figure 15-1B).

    2. The colonic epithelium undergoes a transition at the pectinate line to a nonkeratinized stratified squamous epithelium (Figure 15-1C).

    3. The upper anal canal is derived embryologically from the **hindgut** (Table 15-1).

B. **The lower anal canal** is lined by a keratinized stratified squamous epithelium (Figure 15-1D). It is derived embryologically from the **proctodeum** (see Table 15-1).

II. MUCOSA of the large intestine is lined by:

A. Surface absorptive cells

B. Goblet cells

C. M cells

III. INTESTINAL GLANDS contain:

A. Stem cells

B. Enteroendocrine cells

IV. GUT-ASSOCIATED LYMPHATIC TISSUE (GALT) is prominent.

V. REPAIR (REGENERATION). Stem cells have a high rate of mitosis and replace surface absorptive cells and goblet cells every 5–6 days.

VI. CLINICAL CONSIDERATIONS

A. **Hirschsprung disease (colonic aganglionosis)** is a congenital defect that results from the failure of neural crest cells to form the myenteric plexus within the sigmoid colon and rectum. This results in a loss of peristalsis in the colon segment **distal** to the normal innervated colon. Patients present with fecal retention and abdominal distention.

B. **Familial adenomatous polyposis coli (FAPC)** is the archetype of adenomatous polyposis syndromes in which patients develop 500–2000 polyps (Figure 15-2) that carpet the mucosal surface of the colon and invariably become malignant.

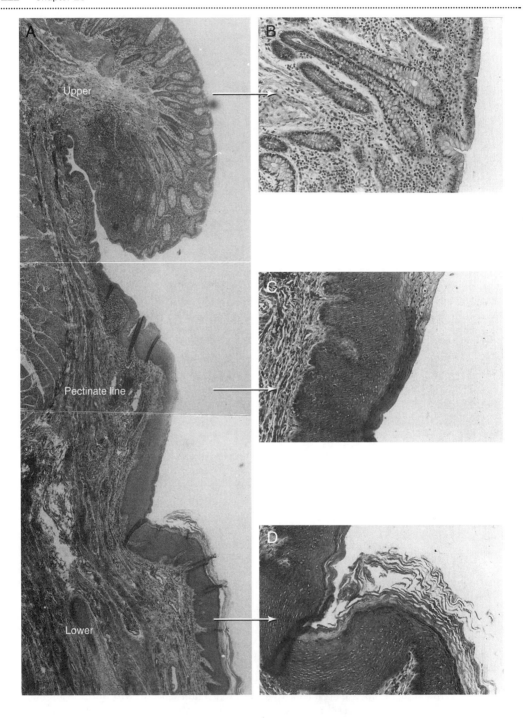

Figure 15-1. (A) Division of the upper and lower anal canal by the *pectinate line*. (B) Typical simple columnar (colonic) epithelium arranged as intestinal glands lining the upper anal canal. (C) Transition of the colonic epithelium at the pectinate line to a nonkeratinized stratified squamous epithelium. (D) Keratinized stratified squamous epithelium lining the lower anal canal.

Table 15-1
Dual Embryologic Origin of the Upper and Lower Anal Canal

Upper Anal Canal (Derived from the Hindgut)	Lower Anal Canal (Derived from the Proctodeum)
Venous drainage is by the superior rectal vein, which drains into the portal vein. Varicosities of the superior rectal vein are called **internal hemorrhoids.**	Venous drainage is by the inferior rectal vein, which drains into the inferior vena cava. Varicosities of the inferior rectal vein are called **external hemorrhoids.**
Tumors drain to **deep** lymphatic nodes (not palpable).	Tumors will drain to **superficial** lymphatic nodes (palpable).
Sensory innervation is for stretch sensation. No pain sensation is present. Therefore, internal hemorrhoids or tumors in this area will not be accompanied by patient complaints of pain.	Sensory innervation is for pain, temperature, and touch. Therefore, external hemorrhoids or tumors in this area will be accompanied by patient complaints of pain.
Motor innervation involves autonomic control of the internal anal sphincter (smooth muscle).	Motor innervation involves voluntary control of the external anal sphincter (skeletal muscle).

1. FAPC accounts for approximately 1% of all colorectal cancer cases and involves a mutation in the **adenomatous polyposis coli (APC) anti-oncogene.**
   a. The **progression from a small polyp to a large polyp** is associated with a mutation in the *ras* **proto-oncogene.**
   b. The **progression from a large polyp to metastatic carcinoma** is associated with mutations in the **DCC anti-oncogene** (deleted in colon carcinoma) and the **p53 anti-oncogene.**
2. **Gardner syndrome** is a variation of FAPC in which patients have adenomatous polyps and multiple osteomas.
3. **Turcot syndrome** is a variation of FAPC in which patients have adenomatous polyps and gliomas.

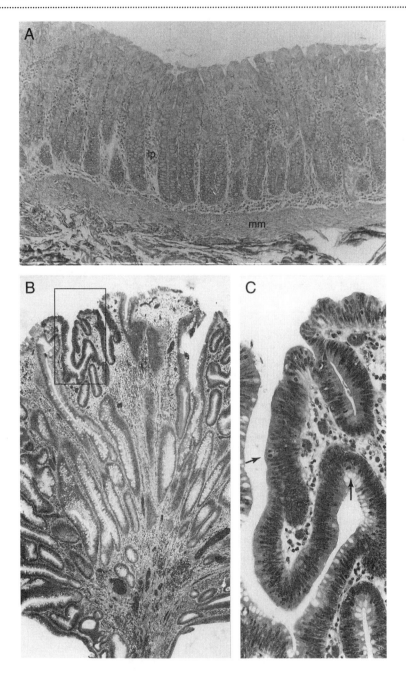

Figure 15-2.   (A) Light micrograph of normal colon. The mucosa shows typical simple columnar (colonic) epithelium arranged as intestinal glands, lamina propria (*lp*), and muscularis mucosa (*mm*). Note the straight, regular arrangement of the intestinal glands that terminate with the basement membrane intact at the muscularis mucosa. (B, C) Light micrograph of an adenomatous polyp. A polyp is a tumorous mass that extends into the lumen of the colon. Note the convoluted, irregular arrangement of the intestinal glands with the basement membrane intact. The epithelium is transformed into a pseudostratified epithelium with mitotic figures apparent (*arrows*; C is a high magnification of the boxed area in B). (B,C From East Carolina University, School of Medicine, Department of Pathology slide collection.)

C. **Adenocarcinomas** (Figure 15-3) account for 98% of all cancers in the large intestine.

    1. Mutations in the **hereditary nonpolyposis colorectal cancer (HNPCC) gene,** which codes for a DNA repair enzyme, have been implicated in some cases.

    2. Adenocarcinomas are characterized clinically by fatigue, weakness, change in bowel habits, weight loss, and iron-deficiency anemia. In fact, it is a clinical maxim that iron-deficiency anemia in an older man means adenocarcinoma of the colon until shown otherwise.

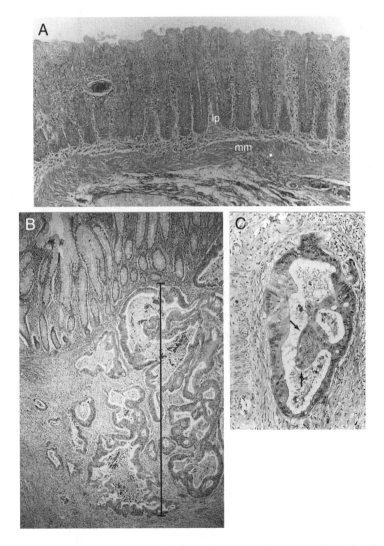

Figure 15-3. (A) Light micrograph of normal colon. The mucosa shows typical simple columnar (colonic) epithelium arranged as intestinal glands, lamina propria (*lp*), and muscularis mucosa (*mm*). Note the straight, regular arrangement of the intestinal glands that terminate with the basement membrane intact at the muscularis mucosa. (B, C) Light micrograph of an adenocarcinoma of the colon. Note the convoluted, irregular arrangement of the intestinal glands that have breached the basement membrane to extend deep into the submucosa and/or muscularis externa (*bracket*). The epithelium is transformed into a pseudostratified epithelium that grows in a disorderly pattern extending into the lumen of the gland (*arrows*; C is a high magnification of a typical area in B). (From East Carolina University, School of Medicine, Department of Pathology slide collection.)

16

Liver

I. HEPATOCYTES

A. Contents include the Golgi complex, rough and smooth endoplasmic reticulum (rER and sER), mitochondria, lysosomes, peroxisomes, lipids, and glycogen.

B. Functions of hepatocytes include the following:

1. Hepatocytes convert ammonium to urea.

2. They form and secrete bile.

3. They conjugate bilirubin.
  a. Bilirubin (water-insoluble) is derived from the breakdown of hemoglobin by macrophages and Kupffer cells.
  b. Bilirubin is endocytosed by hepatocytes and conjugated to glucuronide by glucuronyltransferase in the sER to form **bilirubin-glucuronide** (water soluble), which is secreted into bile canaliculi and excreted in feces.

4. Hepatocytes maintain blood glucose levels by glucose uptake and glycogen synthesis.

5. Hepatocytes degrade glycogen to glucose.

6. They perform gluconeogenesis (conversion of amino acids and lipids into glucose).

7. Hepatocytes maintain blood lipid levels by fatty acid uptake, fatty acid esterification to triglycerides in the sER, and combination of triglycerides with protein in the Golgi complex to form **lipoproteins** (Figure 16-1), which include the following:
  a. Very-low-density lipoprotein (VLDL) is rich in triacylglycerides and travels to adipose tissue and skeletal muscle, where the triacylglycerides are hydrolyzed by lipoprotein lipase to fatty acids.
  b. Low-density lipoprotein (LDL) is rich in cholesterol and distributes cholesterol to cells throughout the body that have specific LDL receptors (see Chapter 1; V C).
  c. High-density lipoprotein (HDL) plays a role in the hydrolysis of triacylglycerides in chylomicrons and VLDL by providing **apoprotein C** for the activation of lipoprotein lipase.
    (1) HDL facilitates the flow of excess plasma triacylglycerides and cholesterol back to the liver; therefore, HDL is called **"good" cholesterol.**
    (2) The enzyme lecithin-cholesterol acyl transferase (LCAT) is associated with HDL and converts cholesterol to cholesterol ester (i.e., cholesterol + a fatty acid).

8. Hepatocytes synthesize cholesterol.

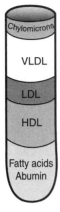

	Density	Triacylglyceride (%)	Cholesterol Free (%)	Esters (%)
Chylomicrons*	<0.94	85	2	4
VLDL	0.94 -1.006	**60**	6	16
LDL	1.019 -1.063	7	**10**	**40**
HDL	1.063 -1.21	5	4	15

*See Chapter 14

Ultracentrifugation

Figure 16-1.   Characteristics of lipoproteins. Lipoproteins are named based on their molecular weight and density separation by ultracentrifugation. Note that very-low-density lipoprotein (VLDL) composition is 60% triacylglycerides, and low-density lipoprotein (LDL) composition is 50% cholesterol.

9. Hepatocytes synthesize plasma proteins (e.g., albumin, fibrinogen, prothrombin).

10. They perform uptake of immunoglobulin A (IgA) and release of secretory IgA into the bile.

11. They perform uptake and inactivation of hormones, lipid-soluble drugs (e.g., barbiturates), and toxins by enzymes in the sER.

12. Hepatocytes metabolize alcohol by using enzymes within peroxisomes.

13. They perform 25-hydroxylation of vitamin D.

14. They secrete α_1-antitrypsin, which is a serum protease inhibitor (α_1-antitrypsin deficiency is an autosomal recessive disorder that results in pulmonary emphysema because tissue-destructive proteases are allowed to act in an uncontrolled manner).

II. KUPFFER CELLS

A. Kupffer cells are macrophages derived from circulating monocytes.

B. They are found in the liver sinusoids.

C. They demonstrate phagocytic activity.

III. LIPOCYTES (FAT-STORING CELLS; ITO CELLS)

A. Lipocytes are found in the perisinusoidal space (space of Disse).

B. They store vitamin A.

C. They may hypertrophy and thereby narrow the diameter of the sinusoid, causing portal hypertension.

IV. CLASSIC LIVER LOBULE (Figure 16-2)

A. The classic liver lobule contains a **central vein** at its center.

B. This lobule also contains six **portal triads** at its periphery, which consists of:

1. A branch of the **hepatic artery**

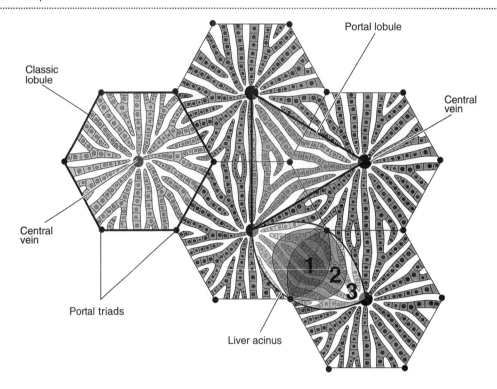

Figure 16-2. Diagram of a classic liver lobule and liver acinus. The classic liver lobule contains a central vein at its center with six portal triads at the periphery. The liver acinus defines three zones (*zones 1, 2, and 3*) based on the location of hepatocytes to incoming blood. Hepatocytes in zone 1 are nearest the incoming blood; hepatocytes in zone 2 are intermediate; and hepatocytes in zone 3 are farthest from the incoming blood. (Reprinted with permission from Henrikson RC, Kaye GI, Mazurkiewicz JE: *NMS Histology.* Baltimore, Williams and Wilkins, 1997, p 292.)

      a. This artery branch carries oxygenated blood.
      b. It contributes 20% of the blood within the liver sinusoids that flows from the periphery to the center of the lobule (i.e., **centripetal flow**).

    2. A branch of the **portal vein**
      a. This vein branch carries nutrient-rich blood.
      b. It contributes 80% of the centripetal flow.

    3. A branch of the **bile duct**
      a. This duct branch carries bile collected from bile canaliculi.
      b. It carries bile that flows from the center of the lobule to the periphery (i.e., **centrifugal flow**).

V. LIVER ACINUS (see Figure 16-2) is divided into **zone 1, zone 2,** and **zone 3** based on the location of hepatocytes to incoming blood. Hepatocytes within each zone have specific characteristics, as indicated in the Table 16-1.

VI. LYMPH

    A. The liver produces 50% of the lymph found in the thoracic duct.

    B. Lymph flows within the space of Disse from the center to the periphery of a liver lobule (i.e., same direction as bile flow).

Table 16-1

Characteristics of Hepatocytes in Liver Acinus Zones

Zones	Characteristics of Hepatocytes
Zone 1	Are exposed to blood high in nutrients and oxygen Undergo necrosis due to chronic hepatitis, primary biliary cirrhosis, bile duct occlusion, and preeclampsia/eclampsia (Note: Hepatic disease is very common in preeclamptic women, and monitoring of platelet count and serum liver enzymes is standard practice.) Undergo necrosis in poisoning due to phosphorus, manganese, ferrous sulfate, allyl alcohol, and endotoxin of *Proteus vulgaris*
Zone 2	Are exposed to blood intermediate in nutrients and oxygen Undergo necrosis due to yellow fever
Zone 3	Are exposed to blood low in nutrients and oxygen Undergo necrosis due to ischemic injury, right-sided cardiac failure, and bone marrow transplantation Undergo necrosis in poisoning due to carbon tetrachloride, cholorform, L-amanitin, pyrrolizidine alkaloids (bush tea), tannic acid, and copper

   C. Lymphatic vessels at the periphery of the liver lobule parallel the branches of the portal vein and ultimately drain into the thoracic duct.

VII. REPAIR (REGENERATION)

   A. Hepatocytes are a relatively stable cell population under normal circumstances (i.e., not under continual renewal).

   B. On partial surgical removal or damage by toxic substances, hepatocytes have a high rate of mitosis.

VIII. CLINICAL CONSIDERATIONS

   A. Viral hepatitis is a term used to describe infection of the liver by a group of viruses that have a particular affinity for the liver, which include the following.

   1. Hepatitis A virus is a self-limiting disease that does not lead to chronic hepatitis or fulminant hepatitis. It is commonly referred to as **infectious hepatitis.**

   2. Hepatitis B virus leads to acute and chronic hepatitis, fulminant hepatitis, and hepatocellular carcinoma. It is transmitted by transfusions, dialysis, and intravenous drug abuse. It is commonly referred to as **serum hepatitis.**

   3. Hepatitis C virus leads to chronic hepatitis, cirrhosis, and hepatocellular carcinoma. It may be the leading cause of chronic hepatitis in the Western world.

   4. Hepatitis D virus leads to hepatitis only in the presence of hepatitis B virus.

   5. Hepatitis E virus is a self-limiting disease that does not lead to chronic hepatitis or fulminant hepatitis. It is transmitted through water.

   B. Primary biliary cirrhosis is caused by a granulomatous destruction of medium-sized **intrahepatic bile ducts,** with cirrhosis appearing late in the course of the disease. It is characterized by **mitochondrial pyruvate dehydrogenase autoantibodies,** the role of which is not clear.

   C. Primary sclerosing cholangitis is caused by inflammation, fibrosis, and segmental dilatation of both **intrahepatic and extrahepatic bile ducts.** It is frequently seen in association with chronic ulcerative colitis of the bowel.

IX. SELECTED PHOTOMICROGRAPHS

A. Electron micrographs of hepatocytes, Kupffer cell, space of Disse, and bile canaliculus and light micrograph of portal triad (Figure 16-3)

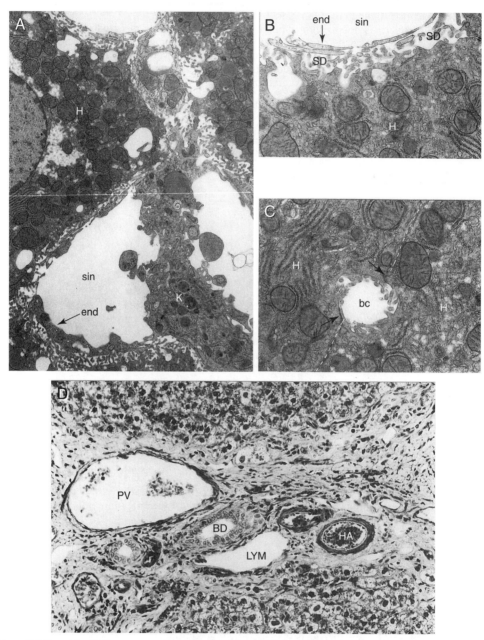

Figure 16-3. (A–C) Electron micrographs of the liver. (A) A Kupffer cell (*K*) is shown within the lumen of a hepatic sinusoid (*sin*). The sinusoid is lined by a discontinuous endothelium (*end*). H = hepatocyte. (B) The apical border of a hepatocytes (*H*) is shown projecting microvilli into the space of Disse (*SD*). The space of Disse is separated from the hepatic sinusoid (*sin*) by a discontinuous endothelium (*end*). (C) Two adjacent hepatocytes (*H*) are shown abutting each other to form a bile canaliculus (*bc*) that is bounded by tight junctions (*arrows*) that serve to contain the bile. (D) Light micrograph of the liver showing the three components of a portal tract: branch of hepatic artery (*HA*), branch of portal vein (*PV*), and branch of bile duct (*BD*). A lymphatic vessel (*LYM*) also is apparent.

B. Light micrograph of normal liver and alcoholic liver cirrhosis (Figure 16-4).

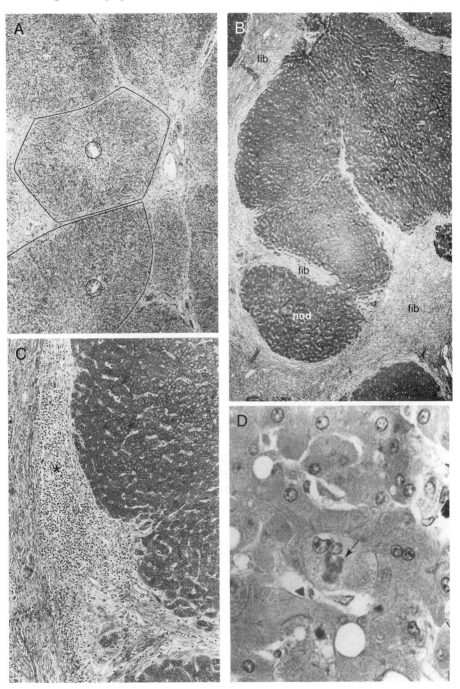

Figure 16-4. (A) Light micrograph of normal liver. The classic liver lobules (*outlined*) with central vein (*circle*) are clearly delineated. (B–D) Light micrographs of alcoholic cirrhosis. (B) Broad bands of fibrous septae (*fib*) are present in alcoholic cirrhosis that bridge regions of the liver from central vein to portal triad and from portal triad to portal triad. This fibrotic activity entraps sections of hepatic parenchyma that undergo regeneration to form nodules (*nod*). (C) Neutrophil, lymphocyte, and macrophage infiltration (*asterisk*) is prominent at the periphery of the liver lobule. (D) Some hepatocytes accumulate tangled masses of cytokeratin intermediate filaments within the cytoplasm known as Mallory bodies (*arrow*). (B–D: Reprinted with permission from East Carolina University, School of Medicine, Department of Pathology slide collection.)

C. Light micrograph of normal gall bladder and cholecystitis (Figure 16-5).

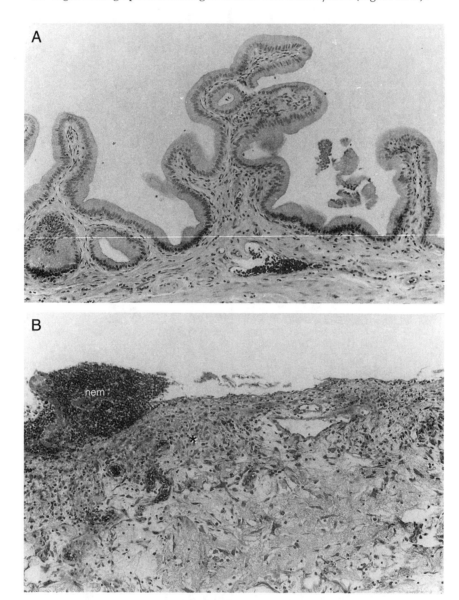

Figure 16-5. (A) Light micrograph of normal gallbladder. Numerous mucosal folds lined by a simple columnar epithelium are shown that project into the lumen of the gallbladder. These mucosal folds flatten out as the gallbladder is distended. At times, the mucosa may penetrate deep into the muscularis externa to form Rokitansky-Aschoff sinuses, which are early indicators of pathologic changes within the mucosa. (B) Light micrograph of cholecystitis. Acute or chronic cholecystitis is generally associated with the presence of gallstones. In this case, the mucosal epithelium is completely obliterated, and there is focal hemorrhage (*hem*) and lymphocyte infiltration (*asterisk*) of the lamina propria. (B: Reprinted with permission from East Carolina University, School of Medicine, Department of Pathology slide collection.)

17

Exocrine Pancreas and Islets of Langerhans

I. EXOCRINE PANCREAS

A. The exocrine pancreas consists of **acinar cells,** which secrete digestive enzymes.

    1. The digestive enzymes secreted by acinar cells include **trypsinogen, chymotrypsinogen, procarboxypeptidase, lipase, amylase, elastase, ribonuclease,** and **deoxyribonuclease.**

    2. Secretion of digestive enzymes is stimulated by **cholecystokinin (CCK)** released by I cells of the small intestine (see Chapter 14; II C).

B. The exocrine pancreas contains a network of ducts that delivers digestive enzymes to the duodenum and secretes **bicarbonate** (HCO_3^-). Secretion of bicarbonate is stimulated by **secretin** released by S cells of the small intestine (see Chapter 14; II C).

II. ISLETS OF LANGERHANS consist mainly of the following cell types (Figure 17-1).

A. Alpha (α) **cells** secrete **glucagon** in response to hypoglycemia to elevate blood glucose, free fatty acid, and ketone levels.

B. Beta (β) **cells** secrete **insulin** in response to hyperglycemia to lower blood glucose, free fatty acid, ketone levels.

C. Delta (δ) **cells** secrete **somatostatin,** which inhibits hormone secretion from nearby cells.

III. INSULIN RECEPTOR AND SIGNAL TRANSDUCTION (Figure 17-2). A receptor (e.g., **insulin receptor**) that activates a chain of cellular events through the **autophosphorylation of tyrosine** is called a **receptor tyrosine kinase** (see Chapter 1; V B).

A. When insulin binds to the insulin receptor, tyrosine kinase autophosphorylates tyrosine residues within the insulin receptor.

B. The phosphorylated insulin receptor subsequently catalyzes the phosphorylation of **insulin receptor substrate-1 (IRS-1).**

C. The phosphorylated IRS-1 plays a role in the following:

    1. Activation and deactivation of many metabolic enzymes

    2. Activation of **phosphatidylinositol 3-kinase (PI 3 kinase)** to produce **inositol 3,4-phosphate** and **inositol 3,4,5-phosphate,** which causes translocation of glucose transporters to the cell membrane

    3. Activation of **Ras protein, Raf protein kinase,** and **mitogen-activated protein**

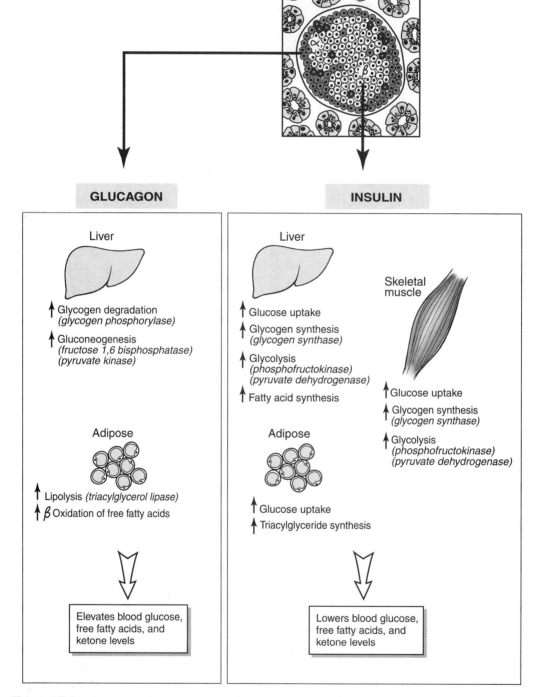

Figure 17-1. The effect of glucagon and insulin on target tissues. The target tissues of glucagon are the liver and adipose. The target tissues of insulin are liver, adipose, and skeletal muscle. The main biochemical pathways and enzymes (*in parentheses*) that are affected by glucagon and insulin are indicated. The alpha (α) cells (*shaded*), beta (β) cells (*white*) and delta (δ) cells (*black*) are shown with the islet of Langerhans. (Figure of islet: Reprinted with permission from Henrikson RC, Kaye GI, Mazurkiewicz JE: *NMS Histology.* Baltimore, Williams and Wilkins, 1997, p 368.)

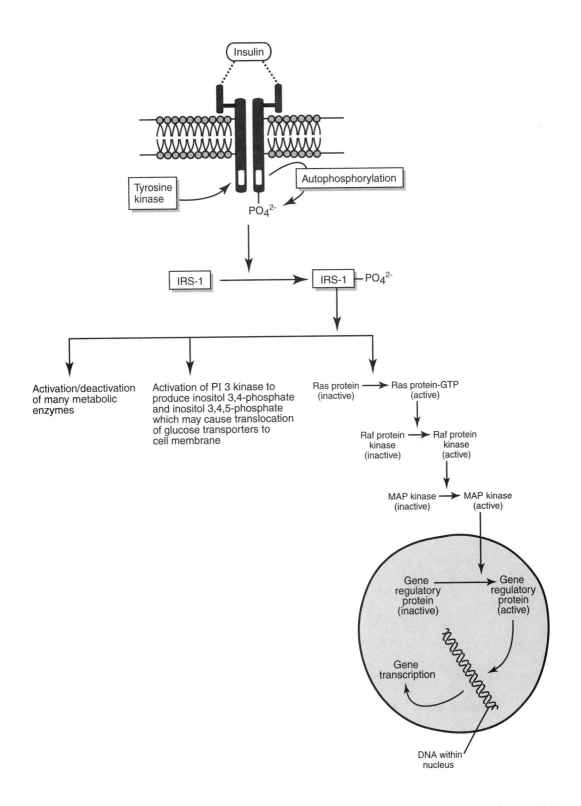

Figure 17-2. The insulin receptor and signal transduction events. *IRS-1* = insulin receptor substrate; *PI 3 kinase* = phosphatidylinositol-3-kinase.

(MAP) kinase, which enters the nucleus, where it activates gene regulatory proteins (e.g., jun) that promote the gene transcription necessary for cell growth and differentiation

IV. CLINICAL CONSIDERATIONS

A. Type 1 diabetes (polygenic)

   1. Characteristics

   a. Type 1 diabetes is marked by **autoantibodies** and an **insulitis reaction** that results in the **destruction of pancreatic beta cells.**

   b. It is characterized clinically by hyperglycemia, ketoacidosis, and exogenous insulin dependence. Long-term clinical effects include neuropathy, retinopathy leading to blindness, and nephropathy leading to kidney failure.

   c. Type 1 diabetes is a **multifactorial inherited disease,** which means that many genes that have a small, equal, and additive effect (genetic component) and an environmental component are involved. If one considers only the genetic component of a multifactorial disease, the term **polygenic** is used.

   2. **Genetic studies** of type 1 diabetes show an association with human leukocyte antigen (HLA) complex loci named **HLA-DR3** and **HLA-DR4** located on the p arm of **chromosome 6 (6p).**

   a. It is hypothesized that genes closely linked to HLA-DR3 and HLA-DR4 loci somehow alter the immune response such that the individual has an immune response to an environmental antigen (e.g., virus). The immune response spills over and leads to the destruction of pancreatic beta cells.

   b. Glutamic acid decarboxylase (GAD_{65}), insulin, and **tyrosine phosphatases IA-2 and IA-2 autoantibodies** are found.

   c. The insulitis reaction is characterized mainly by infiltration of islets by **CD8+ T lymphocytes.**

B. Type 2 diabetes (polygenic)

   1. Characteristics

   a. Type 2 diabetes is marked by **insulin resistance of peripheral tissues** and **abnormal beta cell function.**

   b. Routine screening often detects hyperglycemia, or patient complaints of polyuria lead to detection of type 2 diabetes.

   c. Individuals pass through phases before the onset of frank symptoms, including the following:

   (1) Hyperinsulinemia is present, and euglycemia is maintained.

   (2) Hyperinsulinemia is present, but postprandial hyperglycemia is observed.

   (3) Insulin secretion declines in the face of persistent insulin resistance of peripheral tissues.

   2. **Genetic component.** Type 2 diabetes is a multifactorial inherited disease. At this time, genetic studies of type 2 diabetes show no association with a major susceptibility gene. Instead, type 2 diabetes may involve multiple genes that convey limited degrees of susceptibility.

C. **Monogenic forms of type 2 diabetes.** Genetic studies of family pedigrees prevalent with type 2 diabetes have identified mutations in a single gene. These are **rare** forms of type 2 diabetes.

   1. **Mitochondrial type 2 diabetes** results from a mutation in the **mitochondrial tRNA^{Leu} gene.**

   2. **Maturity onset diabetes of the young (MODY)**

   a. MODY 1 results from a mutation in the **hepatocyte nuclear factor 4α (HNF-4α) gene** located on chromosome 20 (20q). HNF-4α is a transcription factor that is a member of the steroid–thyroid superfamily of nuclear receptors.

   b. MODY 2 results from a mutation in the **glucokinase gene** located on chromosome 7. Glucokinase is an enzyme that catalyzes the conversion of glucose to glucose-6-phosphate and plays a key role in generating the metabolic signal for insulin secretion.

   c. MODY 3 results from a mutation in the **HNF-1α gene** located on chromosome 12 (12q). HNF-1α is a homeodomain transcription factor.

  3. **Leprechaunism** results from a mutation in the **insulin receptor gene.** Leprechaunism is characterized clinically by extreme insulin resistance, growth retardation, dysmorphic facies, and acanthosis nigricans.

D. **Drug treatment of diabetes** involves not only daily insulin injections but also oral glycemic agents, which include the following:

  1. **Sulfonylureas** stimulate insulin secretion.

  2. **Biguanides** (e.g., **metformin**) promote glucose utilization and reduce hepatic gluconeogenesis.

  3. **α-Glucosidase inhibitors (e.g., acarbose, miglitol)** slow down carbohydrate absorption from the intestine.

  4. **Thiazolidinediones** (e.g., **troglitazone, Rezulin**) improve insulin action by activating the **peroxisome proliferator-activated receptor-γ (PPAR-γ),** which modulates a number of genes involved in lipid metabolism.

V. SELECTED PHOTOMICROGRAPHS

A. Normal exocrine pancreas and pancreatitis (Figure 17-3)

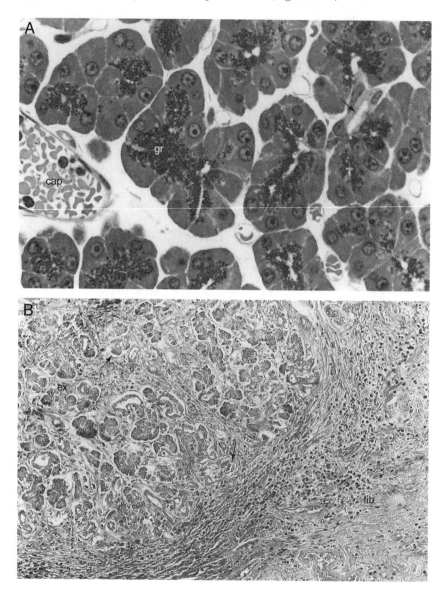

Figure 17-3. (A) Light micrograph of normal exocrine pancreas. Acinar cells containing numerous granules (*gr*) are arranged in clusters. A small capillary (*cap*) and duct (*arrow*) can be observed. (B) Light micrograph of pancreatitis. A large area of exocrine pancreas (*ex*) is shown surrounded by thick fibrous bands (*fib*) that are highly infiltrated with lymphocytes (inflammatory response). Acinar cells undergoing autolysis are shown (*arrows*). Acute pancreatitis is associated in 80% of patients with biliary tract disease or obstruction and alcoholism. The pathologic destruction of the pancreas results from the release of digestive enzymes from acinar cells. (*B:* Reprinted with permission from East Carolina University, School of Medicine, Department of Pathology slide collection.)

B. Islet of Langerhans in normal patient, patient with type 1 diabetes, and patient with type 2 diabetes (Figure 17-4)

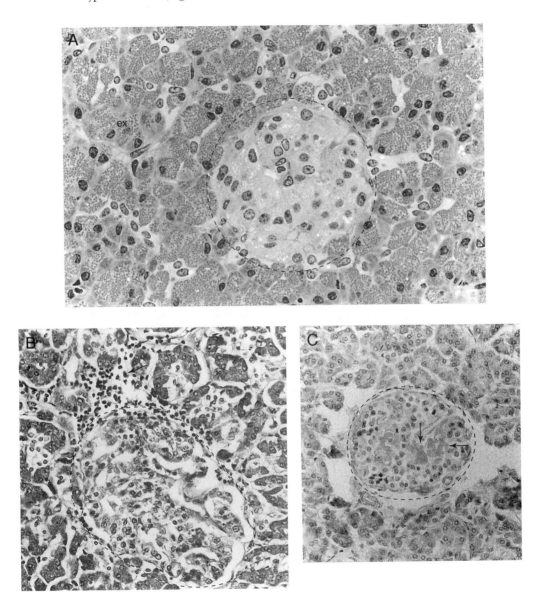

Figure 17-4.   (A) Light micrograph of normal islet of Langerhans. A normal islet of Langerhans (*dotted circle*) is shown surrounded by exocrine pancreas (*ex*). (B) Light micrograph of an islet of Langerhans in a patient with type 1 diabetes. The islet (*dotted circle*) is shown with conspicuous lymphocytic infiltration (insulitis reaction; *arrow*) that probably leads to the destruction of the beta cells within the islet. (C) Light micrograph of an islet of Langerhans in a patient with type 2 diabetes. The islet (*dotted circle*) is shown with conspicuous amyloid (see Chapter 3 V G) deposition (*arrows*). (B, C: Reprinted with permission from East Carolina University, School of Medicine, Department of Pathology slide collection.)

18
Respiratory System

I. CONDUCTION PORTION. This portion of the respiratory system **only conducts air into the lungs.** No blood–air gas exchange occurs in this portion.

A. Contents. The conduction portion consists of the trachea, bronchi, bronchioles, and terminal bronchioles.

1. The trachea and bronchi are lined by a **respiratory epithelium,** which is classically described as a ciliated pseudostratified epithelium with goblet cells that contains the following cell types:

a. Ciliated cells beat toward the pharynx, thereby moving mucus and/or particulate matter to the mouth, where it can be swallowed or expectorated.

b. Goblet cells secrete mucus.

c. Brush cells contain microvilli and have been interpreted as either an intermediate stage in the differentiation to ciliated cells or as a sensory cell because they may be found in association with nerve terminals.

d. Endocrine cells secrete peptide hormones and catecholamines.

e. Basal cells are capable of mitosis.

2. The bronchioles and terminal bronchioles are lined by a simple columnar or simple cuboidal epithelium containing **Clara cells.** Clara cells secrete glycosaminoglycans and contain cytochrome P_{450} to metabolize airborne toxins.

B. Air flow is inversely proportional to airway resistance.

1. Airway resistance is described by **Poiseuille law** as shown in the following equation:

$$R = \frac{8nl}{\pi r^4}$$

where, R = resistance
n = viscosity of inspired gas
l = length of airway
r = radius of airway

Note the strong relationship of r to R. If airway radius (r) is reduced by a factor of 2, then airway resistance (R) is increased by a factor of 16 (2^4), which dramatically reduces air flow.

2. The **medium-sized bronchi** are the main site of airway resistance through the contraction or relaxation of smooth muscle.

a. Parasympathetic stimulation constricts the airways (i.e., reduces r) and thereby increases airway resistance (R).

     b. Sympathetic stimulation or a **sympathetic agonist (e.g., isoproterenol)** dilates the airways (i.e., increases r) and thereby decreases airway resistance (R).

II. RESPIRATORY PORTION. This portion of the respiratory system is where **blood–air gas exchange occurs.**

    A. Contents. The respiratory portion consists of respiratory bronchioles, alveolar ducts, alveolar sacs, and alveoli.

    B. The **alveoli** consists of the following:

        1. Type I pneumocytes are a simple squamous epithelium that line the alveoli. They have no mitotic capacity.

        2. Type II pneumocytes secrete **surfactant,** which is stored as **lamellar bodies.** They have mitotic capacity.

        3. Alveolar macrophages exist in the alveoli.

        4. Alveolar pores (pores of Kohn) are found within the interalveolar septum. They equalize pressure within alveoli and play a significant role in obstructive lung disease by serving as a bypass to aerate alveoli distal to the blockage.

III. SURFACTANT is composed of phospholipids that are enriched in **dipalmitoylphosphatidylcholine** and contain **surfactant proteins A,B,** and **C.**

    A. Surfactant lines the alveoli and **reduces surface tension,** which prevents the collapse of small alveoli (atelectasis), cyanosis, and respiratory distress.

    B. The pressure tending to collapse alveoli is described by **Laplace law** as shown in the following equation:

$$P = \frac{2T}{r}$$

    where, P = collapsing pressure on alveolus
          T = surface tension
          r = radius of alveolus

IV. COMPONENTS OF THE BLOOD–AIR BARRIER

    A. Surfactant layer

    B. Type I pneumocyte

    C. Basal lamina

    D. Capillary endothelial cells

V. REPAIR (REGENERATION)

    A. Basal cells within the respiratory epithelium have mitotic capacity and replace the lining of the conduction portion.

    B. Type II pneumocytes have mitotic capacity and replace both the type I pneumocytes and type II pneumocytes.

VI. CLINICAL CONSIDERATIONS

    A. Respiratory distress syndrome is caused by a deficiency of surfactant, which may occur due to prolonged intrauterine asphyxia, premature birth, or in infants of diabetic mothers.

1. Thyroxine and cortisol treatment increase production of surfactant.

2. Not only is immediate asphyxiation a concern in these infants, but also repeated gasping inhalations can damage the alveolar lining, leading to **hyaline membrane disease.**

B. Bronchogenic carcinoma is classified histologically into the following types:

1. Squamous cell carcinoma is associated with a smoking history, arises in large bronchi, and has a high rate of growth. Well-differentiated forms of squamous cell carcinoma produce **keratin.**

2. Adenocarcinoma is associated with a nonsmoking history. Well-differentiated forms of adenocarcinoma have obvious glandular elements that contain **mucin.**

3. Small cell carcinoma is associated with a smoking history. This highly malignant tumor contains small, oval-shaped cells with neurosecretory granules **(oat cells)** that may produce **ectopic hormones.**

C. Cystic fibrosis (CF) is caused by production of abnormally thick mucus by epithelial cells lining the respiratory (and gastrointestinal) tract. This results clinically in obstruction of airways and recurrent bacterial infections.

1. CF is due to autosomal recessive mutations of the CF gene, which is located on the long arm of chromosome 7 (7q).

2. The CF gene encodes for a protein **called cystic fibrosis transporter (CFTR),** which functions as a **chloride ion channel.**

3. In North America, 70% of CF cases are due to a deletion of three bases that normally code for the amino acid **phenylalanine at position 508,** such that phenylalanine is missing from CFTR.

D. Lung infections

1. *Staphylococcus aureus* produces lung abscesses and is a common secondary infection in rubeola or influenza.

2. *Chlamydia trachomatis* produces pneumonia that is contracted as a newborn infant passes through the birth canal.

3. *Candida albicans* produces pneumonia that is associated with an indwelling catheter and immunodeficiency states.

4. *Coxiella burnetii* is a respiratory pathogen that is commonly found in individuals who have close association with cows, sheep, or goats.

5. *Histoplasma capsulatum* is a fungus that causes an infection characterized by multiple granulomas with calcification in the lung. It is acquired by inhalation of spores and is the most common systemic fungal disease in the midwest United States.

6. *Aspergillus fumigatus* is a fungus that resides in old tuberculous cavities.

7. *Coccidioides immitis* (valley fever) is a fungus acquired by inhalation of spores and is most common in the southwest United States (San Joaquin Valley).

8. *Pneumocystis carinii* is an opportunistic fungus that causes an infection that is a common initial presentation of AIDS.

VII. SELECTED PHOTOMICROGRAPHS

A. Blood–air barrier (Figure 18-1; see IV)

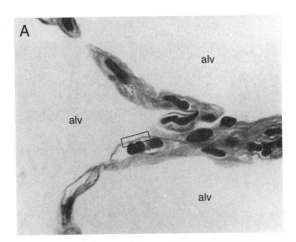

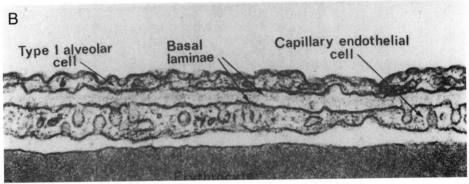

Figure 18-1. (A) Light micrograph of an interalveolar septum. The junction of three alveoli (*alv*) are shown. The area within the box shows the blood–air barrier, which separates the blood (erythrocyte within the capillary) and air within the alveolus. (B) Electron micrograph of *boxed area in* A shows the components of the blood–air barrier: the type I pneumocyte (borders the air interface), the basal lamina, and the capillary endothelial (borders the blood interface). The surfactant layer covering the type I pneumocyte is not shown. Note the histologic layers that air must traverse to get to the erythrocyte. (B: Reprinted with permission from Fawcett DW: *A Textbook of Histology,* 12th ed. New York, Chapman Hall, 1994, p 723. Courtesy of P. Gehr.)

B. Type II pneumocyte (Figure 18-2; see II B 2)

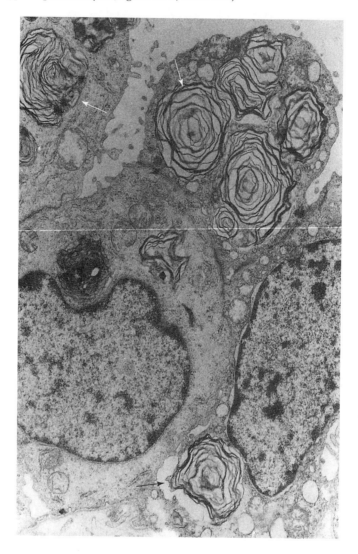

Figure 18-2. Electron micrograph of type II pneumocytes that secrete surfactant. Note the lamellar bodies (*arrows*). (Reprinted with permission from Stahlman MT, Gray ME, Whitsett JA. The ontogeny and distribution of surfactant protein B in human fetuses and newborns. *J Histochem Cytochem* 40 (10):1471–1480, 1992.)

Figure 18-3. (A) Light micrograph of hyaline membrane disease due to respiratory distress syndrome (i.e., deficiency of surfactant). Note the air-filled bronchioles and alveolar ducts that are widely dilated. They are lined by a homogenous hyaline material consisting of fibrin and necrotic cells. In addition, there is atelectasis or collapse of more distal alveoli. (B) Light micrograph of squamous cell carcinoma. Note the irregular nests (*asterisk*) of squamous cell carcinoma. In some nests, keratinization is present (*arrow*). (C) Light micrograph of cystic fibrosis. A bronchus that is filled with a thick mucus and inflammatory cells is shown (*arrow*). Smaller bronchi may be completely plugged by this material. In addition, surrounding the bronchus there is a heavy lymphocyte infiltration (*asterisk*). (Reprinted with permission from East Carolina University, School of Medicine, Department of Pathology slide collection.)

C. Hyaline membrane disease (Figure 18-3; see VI A 1), **squamous cell carcinoma** (see VI B 1), **cystic fibrosis** (see VI C)

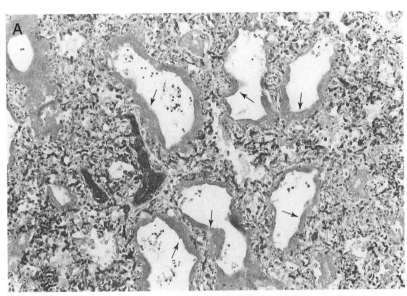

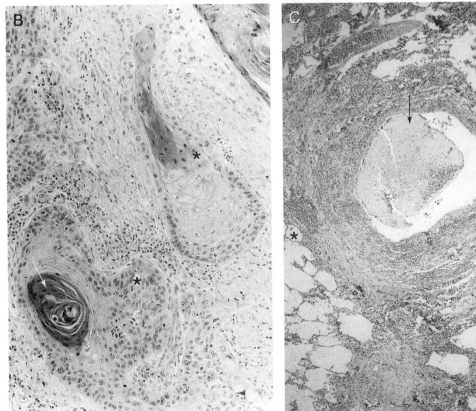

19

Urinary System

I. RENAL (URINIFEROUS) TUBULES (Figure 19-1) are the structural and functional units of the kidney and consist of a **nephron** and a **collecting duct.**

II. NEPHRONS consist of the following:

A. The **renal glomerulus** is a capillary network that receives blood from an **afferent arteriole** (major site of autoregulation of blood flow) and is drained by an **efferent arteriole.**

    1. It contains a **mesangium** (extracellular matrix between capillaries) and **mesangial cells,** which have a phagocytic function, as well as receptors for angiotensin II and atrial natriuretic peptide.

    2. It contains **juxtaglomerular (JG) cells.**

B. The **renal capsule (Bowman's capsule)** consists of **simple squamous epithelium (parietal layer)** that lines the outer wall and **podocytes (visceral layer)** that cover the capillary network. It contains the **urinary space,** which is between the parietal and visceral layers and is continuous with the lumen of the proximal convoluted tubule.

C. **Proximal convoluted tubule** consists of simple cuboidal epithelium with a brush border (microvilli), apical endocytic vesicles, lateral interdigitations, and basal infoldings [with numerous mitochondria and Na+-K+-adenosine triphosphatase (ATPase)].

D. Loop of Henle

    1. The **proximal straight tubule (PST)** is similar in morphology to the proximal convoluted tubule.

    2. The **descending thin limb (DTL)** consists of simple squamous epithelium.

    3. The **ascending thin limb (ATL)** consists of simple squamous epithelium.

    4. The **distal straight tubule (DST)** is similar in morphology to the distal convoluted tubule. In the region of the afferent and efferent arterioles, the DST contains specialized **macula densa** cells.

E. The **distal convoluted tubule** consists of simple cuboidal epithelium with basal infoldings (with numerous mitochondria and Na^+-K^+-ATPase). **Principal cells** and **intercalated cells** have been specifically described within the epithelium.

F. The **connecting tubule** consists of **principal cells** and **intercalated cells.**

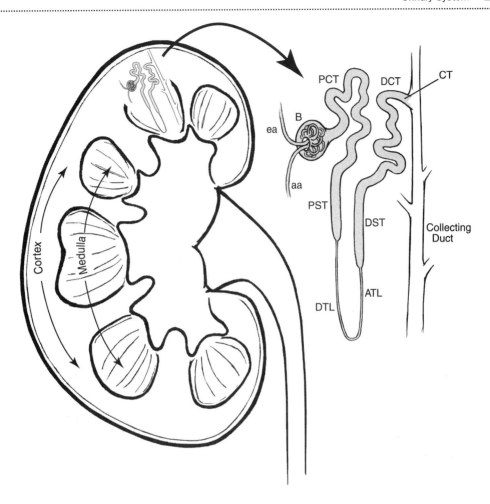

Figure 19-1.   Diagram of an uriniferous tubule. The uriniferous tubule is the structural and functional unit of the kidney. It consists of a nephron and collecting duct. The nephron (*shaded area*) consists of the renal glomerulus formed by the afferent arteriole (*aa*) and efferent arteriole (*ea*), renal (Bowman's) capsule (B), proximal convoluted tubule (*PCT*), proximal straight tubule (*PST*), descending thin limb (*DTL*), ascending thin limb (*ATL*), distal straight tubule (*DST*), distal convoluted tubule (*DCT*), and connecting tubule (*CT*). Note that a distinguishing feature of the kidney cortex is the presence of renal glomeruli, proximal convoluted tubule, and distal convoluted tubule. (Modified and reprinted with permission from Henrikson RC, Kaye GI, Mazurkiewicz JE: *NMS Histology.* Baltimore, Williams and Wilkins, 1997, p 327.)

III. THE COLLECTING DUCT consists of **principal cells** and **intercalated cells.**

IV. FILTRATION BARRIER

    A. Components

        1. **Capillary endothelium** contains continuous, fenestrated (without diaphragms) capillaries.

        2. **Basal lamina** contains **fibronectin, laminin, type IV collagen, and heparan sulfate** (most important in maintaining the negative charge).

3. Filtration slits of podocytes. Podocytes have processes called **pedicles** that con-tact the basal lamina. The gaps between the pedicles are called **filtration slits.**

B. Functions of the filtration barrier include the following:

1. It prevents passage of red blood cells, leukocytes, and platelets.

2. It restricts passage of negatively charged substances (charge filter) and proteins >70,000 d (size filter).

3. It permits passage of water, ions, and other small molecules.

4. It forms an ultrafiltrate of blood.

V. THE JUXTAGLOMERULAR COMPLEX plays a role in blood pressure regulation.

A. Components

1. JG cells are modified smooth muscle cells of the afferent arteriole that secrete **renin** (a proteolytic enzyme).

2. Extraglomerular mesangial cells (Lacis cells) are located between the afferent and efferent arterioles that have receptors for angiotensin II and atrial natriuretic peptide.

3. Macula densa cells are located in the wall of the distal straight tubule (DST) that monitor a decrease in the concentration of sodium ions (Na^+) in the DST fluid.

B. Mechanism of blood pressure regulation

1. An increase in activity of renal sympathetic nerves, a decrease in blood pressure sensed by the afferent arteriole, or a decrease in Na^+ within the tubular fluid sensed by the macula densa cells stimulates JG cells to secrete **renin** into the bloodstream.

2. Renin converts **angiotensinogen** to **angiotensin I.**

3. Angiotensin I is converted to **angiotensin II** (primarily by endothelium of lung capillaries).

4. Angiotensin II causes the following reactions:
  a. Vasoconstriction of arterioles in most organs
  b. Aldosterone secretion from the adrenal cortex (zona glomerulosa), which in-creases Na^+ reabsorption from tubular fluid to blood (water follows) by the cortical collecting ducts (CD) and increases potassium ion (K^+) secretion from blood to tubular fluid by CD
  c. ADH secretion from the neurohypophysis, which increases H_2O reabsorption from tubular fluid to blood by the medullary collecting ducts (CD)

VI. HISTOPHYSIOLOGY (Table 19-1)

VII. THE COUNTERCURRENT MULTIPLIER SYSTEM creates the hyperosmolarity gradient of the interstitial fluid in the kidney medulla, which is crucial for urine concen-tration. The countercurrent multiplier system involves the **loop of Henle,** where tubular fluid flows down the descending limb (proximal straight tubule and descending thin limb) and then back up the ascending limb (ATL and DST); hence the term countercurrent. The differences in permeability of the ascending limb and descending limb (see Table 19-1) establish a small osmolarity difference. However, the countercurrent flow multiplies this small osmolarity difference such that a hyperosmolarity gradient of 300–1400 mOsm is es-tablished; hence the term multiplier.

Table 19-1
Function of Various Renal Tubules

Tubules*	Functions
PCT (major reabsorber)	Reabsorption from tubular fluid to blood 65% of Na^+, 55% of K^+, 80% of Ca^{2+}, 85% of PO_4^{2-}, 65% of H_2O, 80% of HCO_3^-, 50% of urea, glucose, amino acids, proteins (hormones and plasma proteins are endocytosed and lysosomally degraded to amino acids), water-soluble vitamins (B complex, C), lactate, ketones (β-hydroxybutyrate, acetoacetate), Kreb cycle intermediates Secretion from blood to tubular fluid Organic cations (e.g., acetylcholine, creatinine, dopamine, epinephrine, atropine, isoproterenol, cimetidine, morphine) Organic anions [e.g., bile salts, fatty acids, para-aminohippurate, hydroxybenzoates, acetazolamide, chlorothiazide, penicillin, salicylates, sulfonamides, urate (gout)] Inorganic cations: H^+, $NH_4{}^+$
Loop of Henle **PST**	Reabsorption from tubular fluid to blood 5% H_2O
DTL	Reabsorption from tubular fluid to blood 5% H_2O
ATL (impermeable to H_2O)	Reabsorption from tubular fluid to blood 10% of Na^+
DST (impermeable to H_2O)	Reabsorption from tubular fluid to blood 15% of Na^+, 30% of K^+, 10% of Ca^{2+}, 10% of HCO_3^- Secretion from blood to tubular fluid H^+
DCT **CT** **Cortical CD (aldosterone sensitive)** **Medullary CD (ADH sensitive)**	Reabsorption from tubular fluid to blood 10% of Na^+, K^+ (depending on dietary intake), 10% of Ca^{2+}, 5%–25% H_2O (depending on water loading or dehydration conditions), 10% of HCO_3^-, 10% of urea by medullary CD Secretion from blood to tubular fluid K^+ (depending on dietary intake) and H^+

PCT = proximal convoluted tubule; *PST* = proximal straight tubule; *DTL* = descending thin limb; *ATL* = ascending thin limb; *DST* = distal straight tubule; *DCT* = distal convoluted tubule; *CT* = connecting tubule; *CD* = collecting duct; *ADH* = antidiuretic hormone.

VIII. THE COUNTERCURRENT EXCHANGER SYSTEM maintains the hyperosmolarity gradient of the interstitial fluid in the kidney medulla, which is crucial for urine concentration. The countercurrent exchanger system involves the **vasa rectae** (capillaries), which form a hairpin loop in which blood flows down the descending side of the loop and then back up the ascending side of the loop; hence the term countercurrent. If the kidney were supplied by an ordinary capillary bed (i.e., no hairpin loop), sodium and chloride ions would diffuse into the capillaries and water would diffuse out of the capillaries, thereby destroying the hyperosmolarity gradient. This is exactly what happens as blood flows down the descending side of the loop, but then the process is reversed or exchanged as blood flows up the ascending side of the loop; hence the term exchanger.

IX. GLOMERULAR FILTRATION RATE (GFR). Inulin (a polysaccharide) can be used to calculate GFR because inulin is freely filterable at the glomerulus, it is not reabsorbed from tubular fluid to blood, and it is not secreted from blood to tubular fluid.

A. The calculation of GFR is given by the following equation:

$$GFR = \frac{U_{In}\,V}{P_{In}} = 180 \text{ L/day or } 7.5\text{L/hr or } 125 \text{ ml/min}$$

where, U_{In} = urine concentration of inulin
V = volume of urine per unit time
P_{In} = arterial plasma concentration of inulin

B. Although inulin gives an accurate measurement of GFR, inulin is not convenient to use clinically. It is more convenient to use **arterial plasma concentration of creatinine (P_{Cr})** as an estimate of GFR because P_{Cr} and GFR are related by the graph in Figure 19-2.

   1. A **normal** patient will have a P_{Cr} of 10 mg/L, indicating a normal GFR of 180 L/day.

   2. A patient with **kidney disease** will have a P_{Cr} of 20 mg/L, indicating an abnormally low GFR of 90 L/day.

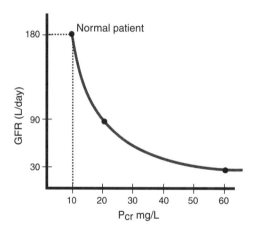

Figure 19-2. Glomerular filtration rate (GFR) compared with arterial plasma concentration of creatinine (P_{Cr}) in a normal patient and in a patient with kidney disease.

X. CLEARANCE is the volume of plasma from which a substance is completely cleared by the kidneys per unit time. The clearance of inulin (C_{In}) is used as a benchmark because inulin is not reabsorbed or secreted by the kidney tubules. Therefore, the C_{In} = GFR = 180 L/day.

A. If clearance of substance X (C_X) is greater than C_{In}, then kidney tubule secretion has occurred. This is another way of saying that if the excreted mass is greater than the filtered mass, **tubular secretion** must have occurred.

B. If clearance of substance Y (C_Y) is less than C_{In}, then kidney tubule reabsorption has occurred. This is another way of saying that if the excreted mass is less than the filtered mass, **tubular reabsorption** must have occurred.

$$C_{creatinine} = 200 \text{ L/day; creatinine is secreted}$$

$$\mathbf{C_{inulin} = 180 \text{ L/day} = GFR}$$

$$C_{urea} = 90 \text{ L/day; 50\% of filtered urea is reabsorbed}$$

$$C_{glucose} = 0 \text{ L/day; 100\% of filtered glucose is reabsorbed}$$

XI. CLINICAL CONSIDERATIONS

A. **Alport syndrome (hereditary nephritis)** is a genetic defect involving the absence of type IV collagen. It results in renal failure and deafness because type IV collagen is an integral component of both the glomerular basal lamina and the tectorial membrane of the inner ear.

B. **Diabetic nephropathy** is characterized by nodular masses of mesangium (Kimmelstiel-Wilson masses) within the renal glomerulus and by hyaline thickening of the glomerular basal lamina.

C. **Renal adenocarcinoma** accounts for 90% of kidney cancers in adults.

1. Renal adenocarcinoma arises from renal tubular epithelium.

2. **Diagnostic features** include costovertebral pain, palpable masses, and hematuria. This tumor generally metastasizes widely (e.g., lung, bones) before any local symptoms or signs are present.

3. It is found in approximately 70% of patients with **von Hippel-Lindau (VHL) syndrome** (i.e., hemangioblastomas of the central nervous system and retina). VHL syndrome is due to a mutation of the **VHL gene** located on the short arm of chromosome 3 (3p) that codes for a tumor suppressor protein probably involved in signal transduction.

XII. SELECTED PHOTOMICROGRAPHS

A. Kidney cortex and kidney medulla (Figure 19-3)

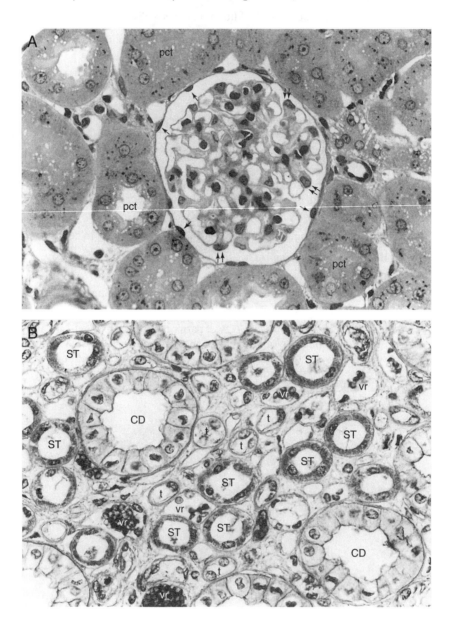

Figure 19-3. (A) Light micrograph of kidney cortex. A renal glomerulus (a capillary network) is shown along with the parietal layer of Bowman's capsule (*arrow*) and visceral layer of Bowman's capsule (podocytes; *double arrows*). PCT = proximal convoluted tubules. (B) Light micrograph of kidney medulla. Cross-sections of various kidney tubules and vasa rectae are shown. *CD* = collecting duct; *ST* = proximal or distal straight tubule; *t* = descending of ascending thin loop of Henle; *vr* = vasa rectae.

B. Podocytes and Na+-K+-ATPase localization (Figure 19-4)

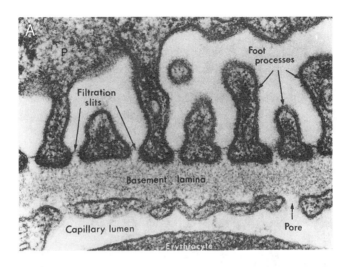

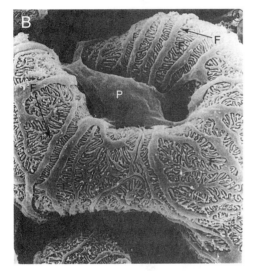
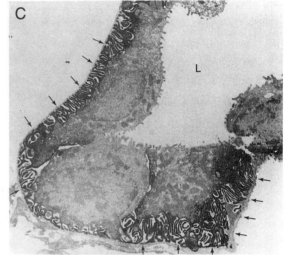

Figure 19-4.   (A) Electron micrograph of the renal glomerulus. A podocyte (P) with its foot processes is adjacent to the basement lamina. Note the *filtration slits* and the *pore* within the endothelial cell of the renal capillary. (Courtesy of D. Friend, Brigham and Womens Hospital, Boston, Massachusetts.) (B) Scanning electron micrograph of the renal glomerulus. A podocyte (P) and foot processes (F) are shown. [Reprinted with permission from Andrews P: Morphological alterations of the glomerular (visceral) epithelium in response to pathological and experimental situations. *J Electron Microsc Tech* 9(2):115, 1988. © 1988, John Wiley & Sons, Inc. Reprinted by permission of Wiley-Liss, Inc., a division of John Wiley & Sons, Inc.] (C) Electron micrograph of a kidney tubule immunocytochemically stained with a monoclonal antibody against the alpha subunit of Na+-K+-ATPase. Basal infoldings (*arrows*) stain (dark black) immunocytochemically positive for Na+-K+-ATPase. L = lumen. [Reprinted with permission from Kashgarian M: Identification of molecules in the kidney utilizing immunocytochemistry. *J Electron Microsc Tech* 9(3):265, 1988. © 1988, John Wiley & Sons, Inc. Reprinted by permission of Wiley-Liss, Inc., a division of John Wiley & Sons, Inc.]

C. Juxtaglomerular apparatus (Figure 19-5)

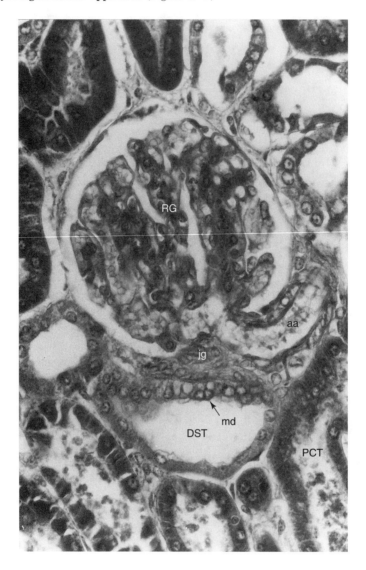

Figure 19-5.   Light micrograph of the juxtaglomerular apparatus. A renal glomerulus (*RG*) and afferent arteriole (*aa*) are shown along with the juxtaglomerular cells (*jg*), which secrete renin. A distal straight tubule (*DST*) can be observed with associated macula densa cells (*md*),which monitor a decrease in the concentration of sodium ions in the DST tubular fluid. A proximal convoluted tubule (*PCT*) also is shown.

D. Wilms tumor and adult polycystic kidney disease (Figure 19-6)

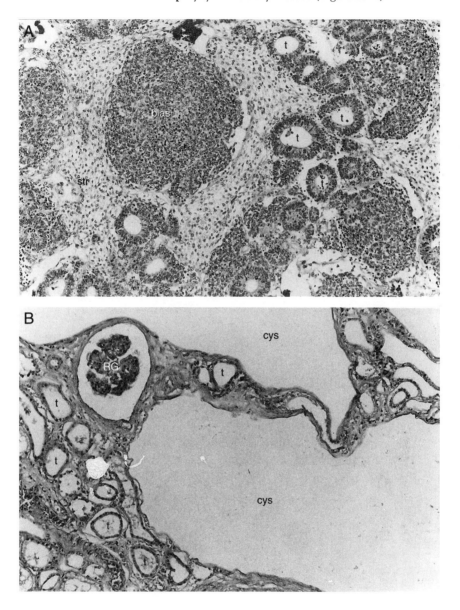

Figure 19-6.   (A) Light micrograph of Wilms tumor. Wilms tumor is a very common primary renal tumor in children. It is characterized histologically by recognizable attempts to recapitulate embryonic development of the kidney. In this regard, the following three components are seen: (1) metanephric blastema elements (*blas*) consisting of clumps of small, tightly-packed embryonic cells, (2) stromal elements (*str*), and (3) epithelial elements generally in the form of abortive attempts at forming tubules (*t*) or glomeruli. (B) Light micrograph of adult polycystic kidney disease (APKD). Large, fluid cysts (*cys*) are found throughout the substance of the kidney. In between the cysts, some functioning nephrons can be found. APKD is an autosomal-dominant disease with 100% penetrance, which means that all individuals with the abnormal gene will express the disease. APKD is associated in approximately 10%–30% of the patients with a berry aneurysm and subarachnoid hemorrhage. *RG* = renal glomerulus; *t* = renal tubules. (Reprinted with permission from East Carolina University, School of Medicine, Department of Pathology slide collection.)

E. Goodpasture disease and malignant nephrosclerosis (Figure 19-7)

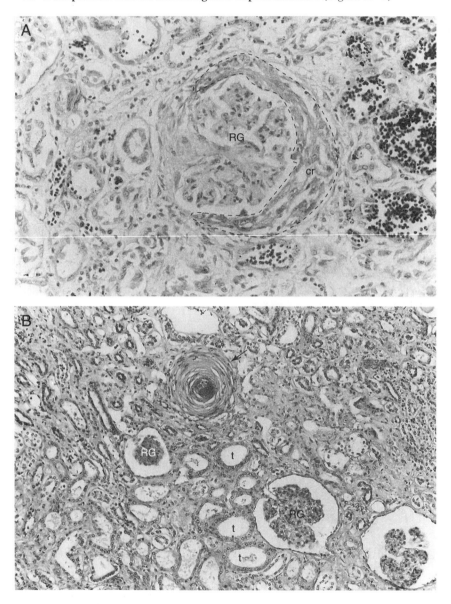

Figure 19-7. (A) Light micrograph of Goodpasture disease. One of the characteristics of Goodpasture disease is the presence of a rapidly progressive (crescentic) glomerulonephritis (RPGN). The RPGN associated with Goodpasture disease is a consequence of basement membrane antibodies. This micrograph shows a renal glomerulus (RG) with a distinctive fibrous crescent (cr; *dotted line*) due to a proliferation of the parietal layer of Bowman's capsule. (B) Light micrograph of malignant nephrosclerosis. Malignant nephrosclerosis is associated with the malignant phase of hypertension. Interlobular arteries and arterioles within the kidney show an intimal thickening due to a proliferation of smooth muscle cells and a concentric layering of collagen. This is called onion skinning or hyperplastic arteriolitis (*arrow*). RG = renal glomerulus; t = renal tubules. (Reprinted with permission from East Carolina University, School of Medicine, Department of Pathology slide collection.)

20
Hypophysis

I. THE ADENOHYPOPHYSIS has three subdivisions, called the pars distalis, pars tuberalis, and pars intermedia.

   A. The **pars distalis** contains important endocrine cells (Table 20-1).

   B. The **pars tuberalis** surrounds the median eminence and infundibular stem of the neurohypophysis. It contains the portal venules of the hypophyseal portal system.

   C. The **pars intermedia** contains numerous colloid-filled cysts (Rathke's cysts) as well as cells that secrete **melanocyte-stimulating hormone (MSH).** It is rudimentary in humans.

II. HORMONAL SECRETION from the adenohypophysis is controlled by hypothalamic neurons and the hypophyseal portal system.

   A. Hypothalamic neurons

      1. Cell bodies are located in the **arcuate nucleus, medial preoptic nucleus,** and **paraventricular nucleus** of the hypothalamus. They synthesize **releasing hormones (RHs)** and **inhibiting hormones (IHs).**

      2. Axons project to the **median eminence,** where axon terminals secrete RHs and IHs into the primary capillaries of the hypophyseal portal system.

      3. RHs and IHs control hormone secretion from the adenohypophysis.

   B. The **hypophyseal portal system** has three components:

      1. Primary capillaries (fenestrated)
         a. Primary capillaries are formed by the superior hypophyseal arteries.
         b. They are located in the median eminence.
         c. They are the site where RHs and IFs are secreted into the bloodstream.

      2. Portal venules
         a. Portal venules are located in the pars tuberalis.
         b. They transport RHs and IHs to the pars distalis.

      3. Secondary capillaries (fenestrated)
         a. Secondary capillaries are located in the pars distalis.
         b. They are the site where RHs and IHs leave the bloodstream to stimulate or inhibit endocrine cells of the adenohypophysis.

   C. Types of RHs and IHs

      1. Thyrotropin-releasing factor (TRF)

      2. Gonadotropin-releasing factor (GRF)

Table 20-1

Characteristics of Endocrine Cells in Pars Distalis

Endocrine Cells	Hormone	Function
Somatotrophs	Growth hormone	Promotes skeletal growth and bone remodeling; hyposecretion causes dwarfism and hypersecretion causes gigantism or acromegaly
Mammotrophs	Prolactin	Promotes growth of the mammary gland during pregnancy and milk secretion in the lactating woman
Thyrotrophs	Thyroid-stimulating hormone	Stimulates triiodothyronine (T_3) and thyroxine (T_4) secretion
Corticotrophs	Adrenocorticotropin (is derived from a large pre-cursor called proopiomela-nocortin)	Stimulates cortisol secretion
Gonadotrophs	Follicle-stimulating hormone	Women: Promotes secondary follicle to Graafian follicle growth Men: Stimulates spermatogenesis and synthesis of androgen-binding protein in Sertoli cells
	Luteinizing hormone	Women: Promotes ovulation (luteinizing hormone surge), formation of corpus luteum, and progesterone secretion Men: Stimulates testosterone secretion from Leydig cells

3. Growth hormone releasing factor (GHRF)

4. Growth hormone inhibiting factor (also called **somatostatin**)

5. Corticotropin releasing factor (CRF)

6. Prolactin inhibiting factor (also called **dopamine**)

III. THE NEUROHYPOPHYSIS (Figure 20-1) receives axonal projections from neurons that have cell bodies that are located in the **supraoptic nucleus** and **paraventricular nucleus** of the hypothalamus.

  A. The cell bodies synthesize **oxytocin,** which causes **milk ejection** (by stimulating myoepithelial cells in the mammary gland to contract) **and uterine contraction during childbirth** (by stimulating smooth muscle cells of the myometrium).

  B. The cell bodies also synthesize **antidiuretic hormone (ADH),** which increases water reabsorption from tubular fluid to blood by the medullary collecting ducts of the kidneys.

  C. Axons project to the neurohypophysis, where axon terminals secrete oxytocin and ADH into the bloodstream.

  D. Axon terminals have large aggregations of neurosecretory vesicles (called **Herring bodies**) containing either oxytocin or ADH (plus a binding protein called **neurophysin**).

  E. **Pituicytes** also are found within the neurohypophysis and may function as glial-type cells.

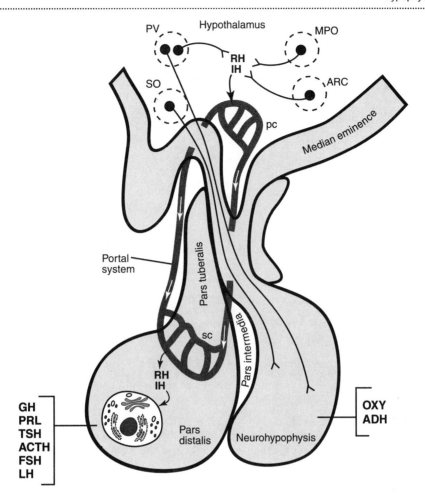

Figure 20-1.   Diagram of the hypophysis [consisting of the adenohypophysis (pars distalis, pars tuberalis, pars intermedia) and neurohypophysis] and hypothalamus. Releasing hormones (*RH*) or inhibitory hormones (*IH*) from the arcuate nucleus (*ARC*), medial preoptic nucleus (*MPO*), and paraventricular nucleus (*PV*) of the hypothalamus enter the primary capillaries (*pc*) of the portal system. RH and IH travel to the secondary capillaries, (*sc*) where they either stimulate or inhibit endocrine cells of the pars distalis. Oxytocin (*OXY*) and antidiuretic hormone (*ADH*) from the supraoptic nucleus (*SO*) and PV nucleus of the hypothalamus travel down axons to the neurohypophysis, where they are secreted through axon terminals into the blood. *ACTH* = adrenocorticotropin; *ADH* = antidiuretic hormone; *FSH* = follicle-stimulating hormone; *GH* = growth hormone; *LH* = luteinizing hormone; *OXY* = oxytocin; *PRL* = prolactin; *TSH* = thyroid-stimulating hormone.

21

Thyroid

I. THYROID FOLLICLES

A. Thyroid follicles are bounded by **follicular** cells and **parafollicular cells.**

B. They are filled with a colloid that consists of **iodinated thyroglobulin.**

II. FOLLICULAR CELLS (Figure 21-1). These cells:

A. Contain **thyroid-stimulating hormone (TSH) receptors**

B. Synthesize thyroglobulin

C. Secrete thyroglobulin into the follicular lumen

D. Take up **iodide** (I^-) from the blood using a $Na^+–I^-$ **cotransporter** and transport it to the follicular lumen

E. Oxidize iodide ($2I^- + H_2O_2 \rightarrow I_2$) using the enzyme **thyroid peroxidase** and **iodinate tyrosine residues in thyroglobulin,** thereby forming monoiodotyrosine (MIT) and diiodotyrosine (DIT), which are then coupled to form triiodothyronine (T_3) and thyroxine (T_4)

F. Are stimulated by TSH to begin **endocytosis** of iodinated thyroglobulin

G. Break down iodinated thyroglobulin into MIT, DIT, T_3, and T_4 through **lysosomal degradation**

H. Deiodinate MIT and DIT using the enzyme **deiodinase** to recycle iodide (I^-); and secrete T_3 and T_4 into the bloodstream, which then circulate bound to **thyroid-binding globulin (TBG).** T_4, which is converted by the liver and kidney into the functionally more potent T_3, accounts for **90%** of the thyroid output; T_3 accounts for **10%** of the thyroid output.

III. FUNCTIONS OF T_3 AND T_4 include the following:

A. Increase the basal rate of oxygen consumption and heat production

B. Increase cardiac output

C. Increase gluconeogenesis and glycogen degradation

D. Stimulate cartilage growth

E. Stimulate endochondral ossification and linear growth of bone

F. Play a crucial role in central nervous system (CNS) development (a deficiency of T_3 and T_4 results in permanent brain damage)

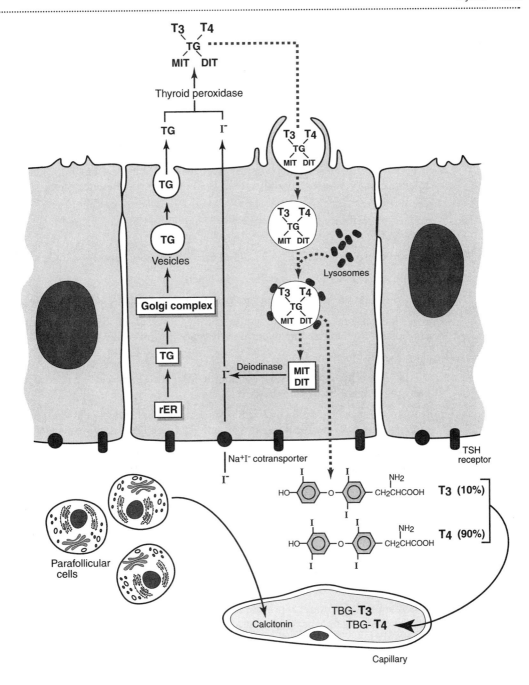

Figure 21-1. Diagram of triiodothyronine (T_3) and thyroxine (T_4) synthesis and secretion by follicular cells. The secretion of calcitonin by parafollicular cells also is shown. DIT = diiodotyrosine; MIT = monoiodotyrosine; TBG = thyroid-binding globulin; TG = thyroglobulin; TSH = thyroid-stimulating hormone.

IV. PARAFOLLICULAR CELLS secrete **calcitonin,** which acts directly on osteoclasts to decrease bone resorption, thereby lowering blood calcium levels.

V. CLINICAL CONSIDERATIONS

A. **Graves disease** is hyperthyroidism caused by a diffuse, hyperplastic goiter.

   1. It is relatively common in women.

   2. It is an autoimmune disease that produces **TSH receptor–stimulating autoantibodies.**

   3. It is characterized clinically by ophthalmopathy (lid stare, eye bulging), heat intolerance, nervousness, irritability, and weight loss in the presence of a good appetite.

B. **Secondary hyperthyroidism** is relatively uncommon and may be caused by a TSH adenoma in the adenohypophysis.

C. **Hashimoto thyroiditis** is the most common cause of goitrous hypothyroidism.

   1. It is relatively common in middle-aged women.

   2. It is an autoimmune disease that produces **thyroid peroxidase autoantibodies.**

   3. It is characterized clinically by goiter and hypothyroidism. In some variants of Hashimoto thyroiditis, only hypothyroidism and no goiter exists.

D. **Primary hypothyroidism**

   1. Primary hypothyroidism is most commonly idiopathic, whereby **TSH receptor–blocking autoantibodies** are present.

   2. It is characterized clinically by low blood pressure, low heart rate, low respiratory rate, reduced body temperature, and myxedema (peripheral nonpitting edema).

E. **Secondary hypothyroidism** is relatively uncommon and caused by a deficiency in the adenohypophysis (low TSH secretion) or hypothalamus [low thyrotropin-releasing factor (TRF) secretion].

F. **Estrogen effect.** The use of **oral contraceptive pills** or the use of **diethylstilbestrol** for treatment of prostatic cancer increases synthesis of TBG.

G. **Diffuse nontoxic (simple) goiter** is an enlargement of the entire thyroid gland in a diffuse manner without producing nodules.

   1. It occurs most commonly in particular geographic areas (called endemic goiter), most often caused by **deficiency of iodine in the diet.**

   2. Wherever endemic goiter is prevalent, endemic **cretinism** occurs. A severe iodine deficiency during fetal development results in growth retardation and severe mental retardation.

H. **Diagnosis.** Table 21-1 shows the laboratory findings used for diagnosis.

Table 21-1

Laboratory Findings Used for Diagnosis of Thyroid Disorders

Disorder	Mechanism	T_4	RT_3U*	FT_4 Index†	TSH
Graves disease	Production of TSH receptor–stimulating autoantibodies	High	High	High	Undetectable
Secondary hyper-thyroidism	TSH adenoma	High	High	High	High
Hashimoto thyroiditis	Production of thyroid peroxidase auto-antibodies	Low	Low	Low	High
Primary hypo-thyroidism	Production of TSH receptor–blocking autoantibodies	Low	Low	Low	Very high
Secondary hypo-thyroidism	Low TSH secretion by adenohypophysis or low TRF secretion by the hypothalamus	Low	Low	Low	Low
Estrogen effect	Oral contraceptives, DES therapy for prostate cancer	High	Low	Normal	Normal

DES = diethylstilbestrol; FT_4 = free thyroxine; RT_3U = resin T_3 uptake test; T_3 = triiodothyronine; T_4 = thyroxine; TRF = thyrotropin-releasing factor; TSH = thyroid-stimulating hormone.

*The resin T_3 uptake (RT_3U) test is not a measure of serum T_3 levels; rather, it evaluates thyroid-binding globulin (TBG) levels via a competition assay between a resin and TBG for radioactive T_3. If TBG levels are low, then more radioactive T_3 will bind to the resin.

†This index is a measure of the true free$_4$ in the serum. It is calculated by multiplying the serum T_4 level by the RT_3U.

VI. SELECTED PHOTOMICROGRAPHS

A. Hashimoto thyroiditis, normal thyroid, and Graves disease (Figure 21-2)

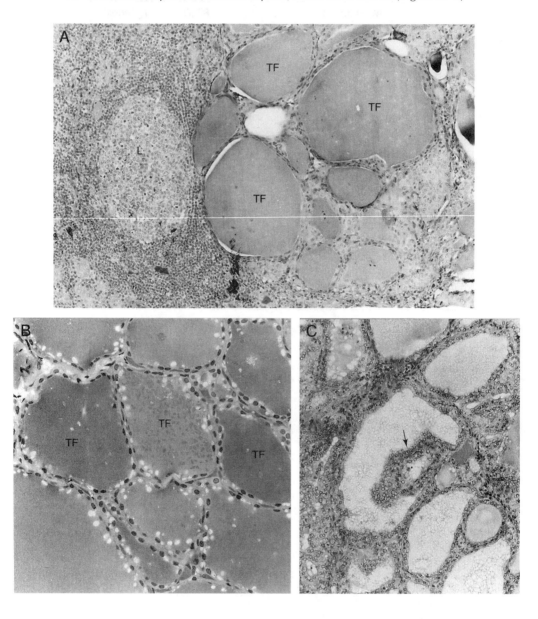

Figure 21-2.   (A) Light micrograph of Hashimoto thyroiditis (*HT*). HT is characterized by a high lympho-cytic infiltration that may form lymphoid follicles with germinal centers (*L*). Normal thyroid follicles (*TF*) also are observed. (B) Light micrograph of a normal thyroid gland showing numerous thyroid follicles (*TF*) contain-ing colloidal material. The follicles are lined by follicular cells arranged as a simple cuboidal epithelium. (C) Light micrograph of Graves disease (*GD*). Graves disease is caused by a diffuse, hyperplastic goiter. The follicu-lar cells are increased in number (hyperplasia) and arranged as a simple tall columnar epithelium. In addition, the follicular cells can form buds that encroach into the colloidal material (*arrow*). (*A and C:* Reprinted with permission from East Carolina University, School of Medicine, Department of Pathology slide collection.)

B. Papillary carcinoma and medullary carcinoma (Figure 21-3)

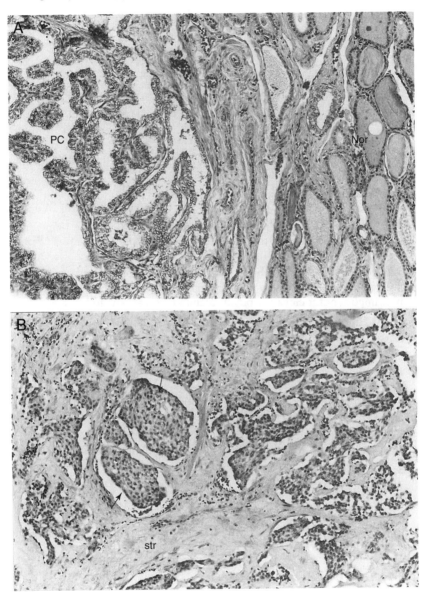

Figure 21-3. (A) Light micrograph of papillary carcinoma (PC). Normal thyroid parenchyma can be observed (*Nor*). PC infiltrates normal thyroid parenchyma and forms elaborate branching papillae that are lined by single-to-multiple layers of follicular cells. The nuclei of follicular cells do not contain nucleoli ("Orphan Annie eyes"). Psammoma bodies sometimes surrounded by calcific lamellations are generally found within the core of the papillae. (B) Light micrograph of medullary carcinoma (MC). MC is an endocrine neoplasm of the parafollicular cells that secretes calcitonin. The parafollicular cells are usually arranged in cell nests (*arrow*) surrounded by bands of stroma (*str*) containing amyloid. Reprinted with permission from East Carolina University, School of Medicine, Department of Pathology slide collection.)

22

Parathyroid

I. CHIEF CELLS secrete **parathyroid hormone (PTH).**

II. OXYPHIL CELLS are distinctly eosinophilic because of the numerous mitochondria within the cytoplasm, but they have no known function.

III. CALCIUM HOMEOSTASIS (Figure 22-1). The body regulates blood calcium levels closely because hypocalcemia results in tetanic convulsions and death. The substances most important for elevating blood calcium levels are the following:

A. PTH

1. PTH acts directly on osteoblasts to secrete interleukin-1 (IL-1), which stimulates osteoclasts to increase bone resorption, thereby **elevating blood calcium levels.**

2. PTH increases kidney reabsorption of calcium from the tubular fluid to the blood, thereby **elevating blood calcium levels.**

3. PTH increases the synthesis of **1α-hydroxylase** in the kidney, thereby **elevating blood 1,25-dihydroxyvitamin D [1,25-(OH)$_2$ vitamin D] levels.**

B. 1,25-(OH)$_2$ vitamin D (see Chapter 5)

1. This substance acts directly on osteoblasts to secrete IL-1, which stimulates osteoclasts to increase bone resorption, thereby **elevating blood calcium levels.**

2. It stimulates absorption of calcium from the intestinal lumen into the blood, thereby **elevating blood calcium levels.**

IV. CLINICAL CONSIDERATIONS

A. Primary hyperparathyroidism (e.g., adenoma, hyperplasia) is characterized by excessive secretion of PTH, leading to hypercalcemia.

B. Malignant tumors (e.g., lung, breast, or ovarian carcinomas) may secrete a **PTH-related protein,** leading to hypercalcemia.

C. Primary hypoparathyroidism (e.g., surgical removal, DiGeorge syndrome, autoimmune destruction) is characterized by the absence of PTH, leading to hypocalcemia.

D. Pseudohypoparathyroidism is a rare condition characterized by abnormal PTH receptors, leading to hypocalcemia, although there are high PTH levels.

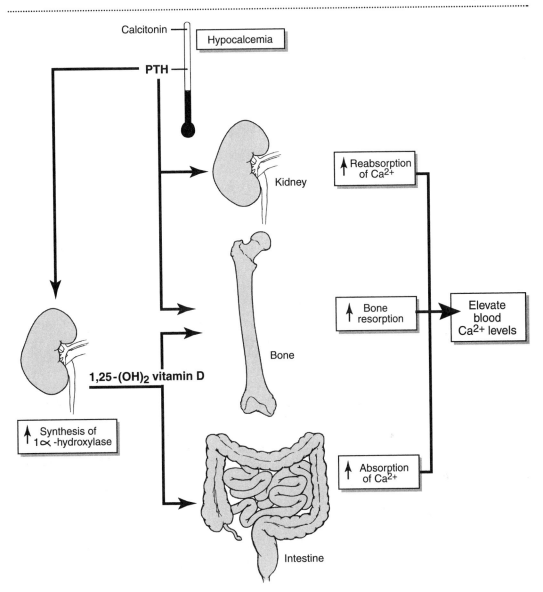

Figure 22-1. Calcium homeostasis. In this diagram, blood calcium levels have decreased, such that *parathyroid hormone* (PTH) is released. PTH and 1,25-(OH)$_2$ vitamin D regulate blood calcium levels by acting on the kidney, bone, and intestine. Blood calcium levels can be depicted on a thermometer such that when blood calcium levels are too high, calcitonin is released. When blood calcium levels are too low, PTH is released.

23

Adrenal

I. CORTEX. Cortical cells of the adrenal gland synthesize and secrete steroid hormones. They have abundant smooth endoplasmic reticulum (sER), mitochondria with tubular cristae, and lipid droplets, which are characteristic of all steroid-secreting cells.

A. Zona glomerulosa (ZG)

1. This region constitutes 15% of the cortical volume.

2. Cells in this region synthesize and secrete **aldosterone.** The secretion of aldosterone is not controlled by **corticotropin-releasing factor (CRF)** and **adrenocorticotropic hormone (ACTH),** which are from the hypothalamus and adenohypophysis, respectively.

3. The **functions of aldosterone** include the following:
   a. Aldosterone increases sodium ion (Na^+) reabsorption from tubular fluid to blood (water follows) by the cortical collecting ducts of the kidneys.
   b. Aldosterone increases potassium ion (K^+) secretion from blood to tubular fluid by the cortical collecting ducts of the kidneys.

4. Aldosterone has a **half-life of 20 minutes** because it is metabolized by the liver and excreted as a glucuronide. Urine levels of **aldosterone 18-glucuronide** are used for diagnostic purposes.

B. Zona fasciculata (ZF)

1. This region constitutes 78% of the cortical volume.

2. Cells in this region synthesize and secrete **cortisol.** The secretion of cortisol is controlled by **CRF** and **ACTH** from the hypothalamus and adenohypophysis, respectively. Abnormally high levels of ACTH (e.g., tumor of adenohypophysis) cause hypertrophy of the ZF. Abnormally low levels of ACTH (e.g., hypophysectomy) cause atrophy of the ZF.

3. The **functions of cortisol** include the following:
   a. Cortisol inhibits glucose uptake in adipose tissue and muscle.
   b. Cortisol stimulates lipolysis in adipose tissue, which forms **glycerol,** used by the liver as substrate for gluconeogenesis, and **fatty acids,** which are metabolized by the liver for energy.
   c. Cortisol stimulates proteolysis in muscle, which forms **amino acids** that are used by the liver as substrate for gluconeogenesis.
   d. Cortisol stimulates gluconeogenesis and glycogen synthesis in the liver (overall the most important metabolic effect of cortisol is the **conversion of fat and muscle protein to glycogen**).
   e. It inhibits bone formation, causing **osteoporosis** by reducing the synthesis of

type I collagen and decreasing the absorption of calcium by the intestinal tract by blocking the action of 1,25-(OH$_2$) vitamin D.

    f. It produces anti-inflammatory and immunosuppressive actions at high concentrations by inhibiting the enzyme **phospholipase A$_2$**, which releases arachidonic acid (a precursor for many immune mediators).

  4. Cortisol has a **half-life of 70 minutes** because it is metabolized by the liver and excreted in the urine as a glucuronide. Urine levels of **17-hydroxycorticoids** are used for diagnostic purposes.

C. Zona reticularis (ZR)

  1. This region constitutes 7% of the cortical volume.

  2. Cells in this region synthesize and secrete **dehydroepiandrosterone (DHEA)** and **androstenedione.** The secretion of DHEA and androstenedione is controlled by **CRF** and **ACTH** from the hypothalamus and adenohypophysis, respectively.

  3. Although DHEA and androstenedione are weak androgens, they are converted to testosterone by peripheral tissues.

  4. The **functions of DHEA and androstenedione** include the following:

    a. In women, DHEA and androstenedione conversion to testosterone is a main source of testosterone. During puberty, DHEA and androstenedione also may serve as substrates for conversion to estrogen.

    b. In men, DHEA and androstenedione conversion to testosterone is of little biological significance because the testes produce most of the testosterone.

  5. DHEA and androstenedione are metabolized by the liver to 17-ketosteroids. Urine levels of **17-ketosteroids** are used for diagnostic purposes.

D. **Synthesis of adrenocortical hormones** uses **cholesterol** as a precursor (Figure 23-1).

E. Clinical considerations

  1. Primary hyperaldosteronism

    a. **Cause.** Elevated levels of aldosterone (i.e., hyperaldosteronism) are commonly caused by an aldosterone-secreting tumor (**Conn syndrome**) within the ZG.

    b. **Symptoms.** Primary hyperaldosteronism is characterized clinically by hypertension, hypernatremia due to increased sodium ion reabsorption, weight gain due to water retention, and hypokalemia due to increased potassium ion secretion.

    c. **Treatment.** It is treated by surgery and/or **spironolactone,** which is an aldosterone receptor antagonist and therefore an effective antihypertensive and diuretic agent.

  2. Cushing syndrome

    a. **Cause.** Elevated levels of cortisol (i.e., hypercortisolism) are commonly caused by an ACTH-secreting tumor within the adenohypophysis (75% of the cases) or adrenal cortical hyperplasia (25% of the cases).

    b. **Symptoms.** Cushing syndrome is characterized clinically by hypertension, osteoporosis with back pain, central obesity, moon facies, and purple skin striae.

    c. **Treatment. Ketoconazole** is an inhibitor of steroid biosynthesis that is used in the treatment of Cushing syndrome.

  3. Congenital adrenal hyperplasia

    a. **Cause.** Congenital adrenal hyperplasia is caused most commonly by mutations in genes for enzymes involved in adrenocortical steroid biosynthesis

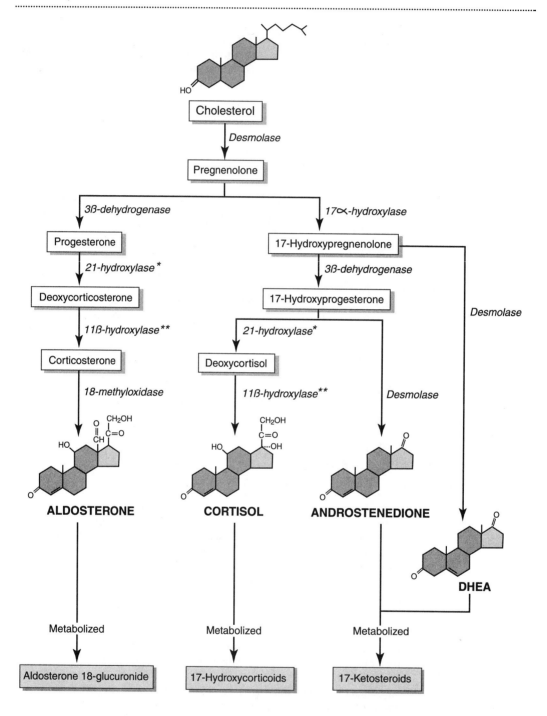

Figure 23-1. Synthesis and metabolism of adrenocortical hormones. Synthesis begins with cholesterol as a precursor. The metabolic urine breakdown products (in *shaded boxes*) are used for diagnostic purposes. 21-hydroxylase (*asterisk*) and 11β-hydroxylase (*double asterisk*) are enzymes involved in congenital adrenal hyperplasia.

(e.g., **21-hydroxylase deficiency, 11β-hydroxylase deficiency**). In 21-hydroxylase deficiency (90% of all cases), there is virtually no synthesis of the aldosterone or cortisol, so that intermediates are funneled into androgen biosynthesis, thereby elevating androgen levels.

   b. Symptoms. The elevated levels of androgens lead to **virilization of a female fetus** ranging from mild clitoral enlargement to complete labioscrotal fusion with a phalloid organ. Because cortisol cannot be synthesized, negative feedback to the adenohypophysis does not occur, so ACTH continues to stimulate the adrenal cortex, resulting in adrenal hyperplasia.

   c. Treatment. Depending on the severity, treatment may include surgical reconstruction and steroid replacement.

4. Primary adrenal insufficiency (Addison disease)
   a. Cause. Addison disease is commonly caused by autoimmune destruction of the adrenal cortex.
   b. Symptoms. It is characterized clinically by fatigue, anorexia, nausea, weight loss, hypotension, and hyperpigmentation of the skin.
   c. Treatment. This condition is managed by steroid replacement therapy.

5. Secondary adrenal insufficiency
   a. Cause. Secondary adrenal insufficiency is caused by a disorder of the hypothalamus or adenohypophysis that reduces the secretion of ACTH.
   b. Symptoms. It is clinically very similar to Addison disease except there is no hyperpigmentation of the skin.

F. Diagnosis. Table 23-1 shows the laboratory findings used for diagnosis. The **dexamethasone suppression test** is based on the ability of dexamethasone (a synthetic glucocorticoid) to inhibit ACTH and cortisol secretion. If the adenohypophysis–adrenal cortex axis is normal, dexamethasone will inhibit ACTH and cortisol secretion by negative feedback.

II. THE MEDULLA contains **chromaffin cells,** which are **modified postganglionic sympathetic neurons.** Preganglionic sympathetic axons (via splanchnic nerves) synapse on chromaffin cells, and upon stimulation cause chromaffin cells to secrete catecholamines, epinephrine, and norepinephrine. There are two types of chromaffin cells:

Table 23-1

Laboratory Findings Used to Diagnose Adrenal Gland Disorders

Clinical Condition	Plasma Levels			
	Aldosterone	**Cortisol**	**Androgens**	**ACTH**
Primary hyperaldosteronism (Conn syndrome)	High	N/A	N/A	N/A
Cushing syndrome				
ACTH tumor	N/A	High	N/A	High
Adrenal hyperplasia	N/A	High	N/A	Low
Congenital adrenal hyperplasia 21-hydroxylase deficiency 11β-hydroxylase deficiency	Low	Low	High	High
Addison disease (primary adrenal insufficiency)	Low	Low	Low	High
Secondary adrenal insufficiency	Normal	Low	Low	Low

ACTH = adrenocorticotropic hormone; *N/A* = not applicable.

A. Epinephrine-containing cells comprise a majority of the chromaffin cells in the medulla and contain small, homogeneous, light-staining granules.

1. All of the circulating epinephrine in the blood is derived from the adrenal medulla.

2. Functions of epinephrine
   a. Stimulates glycogen degradation in the liver, thereby releasing free glucose
   b. Stimulates glycogen degradation in skeletal muscle, thereby releasing lactic acid
   c. Stimulates lipolysis in adipose tissue, thereby releasing free fatty acids
   d. Inhibits glucose uptake in adipose tissue and muscle so that glucose is available for the brain
   e. Inhibits insulin secretion
   f. Affects nonvascular smooth muscle cells

3. Epinephrine has a **half-life of 1–3 minutes** because it is metabolized by the liver and excreted in the urine as free epinephrine, metanephrine, or as a glucuronide. **Urinary free epinephrine** or **plasma epinephrine levels** are used for diagnostic purposes in problems of adrenal medulla function.

B. Norepinephrine-containing cells comprise a minority of the chromaffin cells in the medulla and contain large, electron-dense core granules.

1. The majority of circulating norepinephrine in the blood is derived from the sympathetic nervous system (postganglionic neurons) and brain, with the secretion from the adrenal medulla contributing only a minor portion.

2. Functions of norepinephrine
   a. Stimulates α-adrenergic receptors on vascular smooth muscle cells, thereby causing vasoconstriction in resting skeletal muscle
   b. Stimulates β-adrenergic receptors on vascular smooth muscle cells, thereby causing vasodilation in resting skeletal muscle
   c. Stimulates β-adrenergic receptors on cardiac myocytes, thereby increasing the heart rate
   d. Stimulates eccrine sweat glands, producing emotional sweating
   e. Stimulates apocrine sweat glands, producing pheromones
   f. Plays a role in anxiety states, panic attacks, and depression
   g. Affects nonvascular smooth muscle cells

3. Norepinephrine has a **half-life of 1–3 minutes,** because it is metabolized by the liver and excreted in the urine as free norepinephrine, normetanephrine, a glucuronide, vanillylmandelic acid (VMA), or 3-methoxy-4-hydroxyphenyglycol (MOPEG). **Urinary levels of VMA and MOPEG** are used for diagnostic purposes in problems of the sympathetic nervous system.

C. Dual blood supply

1. The medulla receives venous blood draining the cortex, which has a high concentration of cortisol. The synthesis of **phenylethanolamine-N-methyltransferase** (a key enzyme in the synthesis of epinephrine) is dependent on high levels of cortisol received via venous blood from the cortex.

2. The medulla also receives arterial blood from capsular arteries that pass through the cortex to form a capillary network around the chromaffin cells.

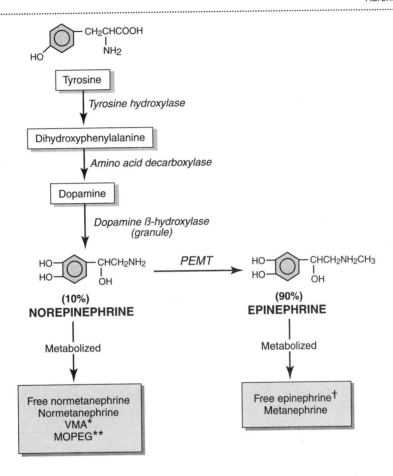

Figure 23-2. Synthesis and metabolism of adrenomedullary catecholamines. Synthesis begins with tyrosine as a precursor. The metabolic urine breakdown products (in *shaded boxes*) are used for diagnostic purposes. Vanillylmandelic acid (*VMA*; *asterisk*) and 3-methoxy-4-hydroxyphenyglycol (MOPEG; *double asterisk*) are diagnostic of sympathetic nervous system function. Urinary free epinephrine (*dagger*) or plasma epinephrine levels are diagnostic of adrenal medulla function. When the adrenal medulla is stimulated, the secretion product is 90% epinephrine and 10% norepinephrine. All of the enzymes involved in catecholamine synthesis are found in the cytoplasm except dopamine β-hydroxylase, which is located within secretion granules. *PEMT* = phenylethanolamine-N-methyltransferase.

> **D.** Synthesis of catecholamines uses **tyrosine** as a precursor (Figure 23-2).
>
> **E. Clinical considerations**
>
> > **1. Pheochromocytoma** is a relatively rare neoplasm that contains both epinephrine and norepinephrine.
> >
> > > **a. Characteristics.** Pheochromocytoma occurs mainly in adults. It is generally found in the region of the adrenal gland but also is found in extra-adrenal sites.
> > >
> > > **b. Symptoms.** It is associated with persistent or paroxysmal hypertension, anxiety, tremor, profuse sweating, pallor, chest pain, and abdominal pain.
> > >
> > > **c. Diagnosis.** Increased urine VMA and metanephrine levels, inability to suppress catecholamines with clonidine, and hyperglycemia are common laboratory findings.

       d. **Treatment.** Pheochromocytoma is treated by surgery or phenoxybenzamine (an α-adrenergic antagonist).

   2. **Neuroblastoma** is a common extracranial neoplasm containing primitive neuroblasts of neural crest origin.

       a. **Characteristics.** Neuroblastomas occur mainly in children. They are found in extra-adrenal sites usually along the sympathetic chain ganglia (60%) or within the adrenal medulla (40%). They metastasize widely.

       b. **Symptoms.** It is associated with **opsoclonus** (rapid, irregular movements of the eye in horizontal and vertical directions; "dancing eyes").

       c. **Diagnosis.** A neuroblastoma contains small cells arranged in **Homer-Wright pseudorosettes.** Increased urine VMA and metanephrine levels are found.

       d. **Treatment** includes surgical excision, radiation, and chemotherapy.

Figure 23-3. (A) Hyperplasia of the adrenal cortex as might be found in Cushing syndrome. (B) Normal adrenal gland showing the normal thickness of the adrenal cortex. (C) Hypoplasia of the adrenal cortex as might be found in Addison disease. All photomicrographs are taken at the same magnification so that the normal and pathologic changes may be compared. C = adrenal cortex; M = adrenal medulla.

III. SELECTED PHOTOMICROGRAPHS

A. Hyperadrenalism (Cushing syndrome), normal adrenal gland, hypoadrenalism (Addison disease) [Figure 23-3]

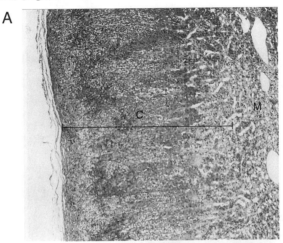

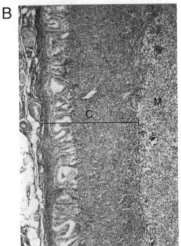

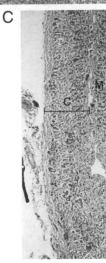

B. Normal adrenal medulla, pheochromocytoma, neuroblastoma (Figure 23-4)

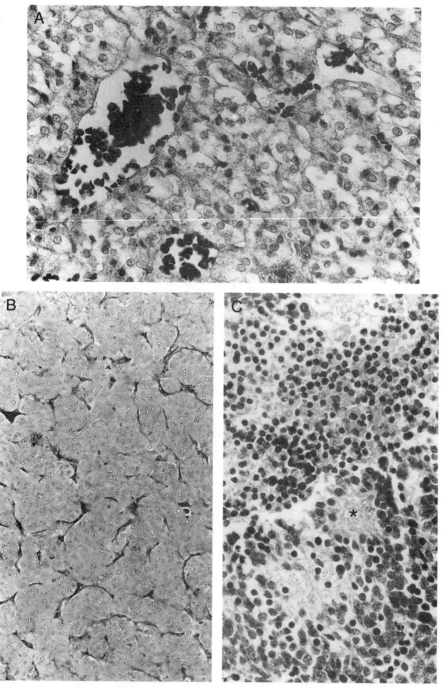

Figure 23-4.   (A) Light micrograph of a normal adrenal medulla showing chromaffin cells and fairly large capillaries. (B) Light micrograph of a pheochromocytoma, which generally appears as a diffuse or nodular hyperplasia. The neoplastic cells are abundant cytoplasm with small centrally located nuclei. The neoplastic cells are separated into clusters by a slender stroma and numerous capillaries. (C) Light micrograph of a neuroblastoma, which is commonly composed of small, primitive-looking cells with dark nuclei and scant cytoplasm. The cells generally are arranged as solid sheets, and some cells arrange around a central fibrillar area, forming Homer-Wright pseudorosettes (*asterisk*).

24

Female Reproductive System

I. ADULT OVARY (CORTEX) contains follicles in various stages of development, including the primordial follicle, primary follicle, secondary follicle, and Graafian follicle. Follicles are composed of an oocyte, follicular cells, and thecal cells (Table 24-1).

II. CORPUS LUTEUM is a temporary endocrine gland. Its formation is **dependent on luteinizing hormone (LH).**

    A. Development. Corpus luteum develops from the granulosa cells and theca interna cells of the Graafian follicle after the secondary oocyte is ovulated through a process called **luteinization** (i.e., cells develop the capacity to produce steroid hormones).

        1. Granulosa lutein cells synthesize and secrete **progesterone.** Progesterone maintains the endometrium of the uterus in the secretory (luteal) phase so that implantation and nutritional support of the blastocyst may occur. **Mifepristone** is a drug that binds to progesterone receptors and blocks progesterone action, thereby inducing early abortion.

        2. Theca lutein cells synthesize and secrete **estrogen** and **estrone.**

    B. Effect of fertilization

        1. If fertilization occurs, the corpus luteum enlarges and becomes the predominant source of steroids needed to sustain pregnancy for approximately 8 weeks. Thereafter, the placenta becomes the major source of the steroids required.

        2. If fertilization does not occur, the corpus luteum regresses and forms a **corpus albicans.**

III. UTERINE TUBES are the site of fertilization.

    A. Uterine tubes are **lined by** two types of cells.

        1. Nonciliated cells secrete a nutrient-rich medium for the nourishment of the sperm and preimplantation embryo.

        2. Ciliated cells have cilia that beat toward the uterus. The rate of ciliary beat is influenced by progesterone and estrogen, and they assist in transport of the preimplantation embryo to the uterus.

    B. Clinical consideration. Salpingitis (acute and chronic) is a bacterial infection (most commonly **gonococcus**) of the uterine tube with acute inflammation (neutrophil infiltration) or chronic inflammation that may lead to scarring of the uterine tube, which predisposes affected women to **ectopic tubal pregnancy.**

Table 24-1
Development of the Ovarian Follicle

Stage of Follicle	Oocyte	Follicular Cells	Thecal Cells
Primordial	Primary oocyte (46, 4N) Arrested in prophase of meiosis I	Squamous cells: 1 layer	Fibroblasts
Primary	Primary oocyte (46, 4N) Arrested in prophase of meiosis I	Granulosa cells: 1 layer	Fibroblasts
Secondary ↓ FSH dependent ↓ Graafian	Primary oocyte (46, 4N) Arrested in prophase of meiosis I Zona pellucida present Secondary oocyte (23, 2N) Arrested in metaphase of meiosis II Zona pellucida present	Granulosa cells: Multiple layers Secrete estrogen by aromatase conversion of androgens from theca interna FSH and LH receptors present	Theca interna: Secrete androgens LH receptors present Theca externa: Fibrous and vascular

FSH = follicle-stimulating hormone; *LH* = luteinizing hormone.

IV. UTERUS

A. **Endometrium** consists of simple columnar epithelium, which invaginates into the endometrial stroma to form **endometrial glands.** The endometrium can be divided into two layers.

  1. **The basal layer** regenerates the functional layer each month during the menstrual cycle. The basal layer is never sloughed off.

  2. **The functional layer** undergoes alterations during the menstrual cycle. The functional layer is sloughed off each month during menses.

B. **The menstrual cycle** is a series of phases that repeats ideally every 28 days.

  1. **The menstrual phase (days 1–4)** is characterized by the **necrosis and shedding** of the functional layer of the endometrium. Spiral arterioles constrict episodically for a few days and finally constrict permanently, resulting in ischemia that leads to necrosis of endometrial glands and stroma. The spiral arterioles subsequently dilate and rupture, resulting in hemorrhage that sheds the necrotic endometrial glands and stroma.

  2. **The proliferative (follicular) phase (days 4–15)** is characterized by the **regeneration** of the functional layer of the endometrium from the devastating effects of the menstrual phase. This phase is **controlled by estrogen** secreted by the granulosa cells of the secondary and Graafian follicle. Epithelial cells and fibroblasts of the basal layer of the endometrium regenerate to form **straight endometrial glands and stroma**, respectively.

  3. **The ovulatory phase (days 14–16)** is characterized by **ovulation** of the secondary oocyte arrested in metaphase of meiosis II that coincides with **peak levels of LH (LH surge).**

4. The secretory (luteal) phase (days 15–25) is characterized by the **secretory activity** of the endometrial glands. This phase is **controlled by progesterone** secreted by the granulosa lutein cells of the corpus luteum. The endometrial glands become modified to **convoluted endometrial glands with secretion product** within their lumen.

5. The premenstrual phase (days 25–28) is characterized by **ischemia** due to reduced blood flow to the endometrium. This phase is **controlled by the reduction in progesterone and estrogen** as the corpus luteum involutes. As the endometrial glands begin to shrink, the spiral arterioles are compressed, thereby reducing blood flow and causing ischemic damage.

C. **Myometrium** consists of smooth muscle cells that are connected by gap junctions and contract on stimulation by **oxytocin** and **prostaglandins** at parturition. The myometrium contains the **stratum vasculare,** which is highly vascular and is the source of the endometrial blood supply.

D. **Perimetrium** consists of connective tissue covered by peritoneal mesothelium.

E. The intricate coordination between the hypothalamus, adenohypophysis, ovaries, and endometrium of the uterus results in the menstrual cycle (Figure 24-1).

F. **Clinical considerations**

    1. **Endometriosis** is the presence of endometrial glands in abnormal locations (e.g., ovary, uterine ligaments, pelvic peritoneum), causing infertility, dysmenorrhea, and pelvic pain.

    2. **Leiomyoma** is a very common benign tumor derived from smooth muscle within the myometrium.

    3. **Amenorrhea** is the absence of menstruation.

        a. **Primary amenorrhea** is the complete absence of menstruation in a woman from puberty.

        b. **Secondary amenorrhea** is the absence of menstruation for at least 3 months in a woman who previously had normal menstruation.

        (1) **Causes.** The most common cause of secondary amenorrhea is pregnancy, which can be determined by assaying urine human chorionic gonadotropin (hCG). Other pathologic causes of secondary amenorrhea include hypothalamic/pituitary malfunction (e.g., **anorexia nervosa**), ovarian disorders (e.g., **ovariectomy**), and end-organ disease (e.g., **Asherman syndrome,** in which the basal layer of the endometrium has been removed by repeated curettages).

        (2) **Diagnosis.** These causes are evaluated clinically by **assaying serum follicle-stimulating hormone (FSH) and LH levels** along with a **progesterone challenge.** Bleeding after a progesterone challenge indicates that the endometrium was primed by estrogen, thereby indicating that the hypothalamic/pituitary axis and the ovaries are functioning normally. The results of such clinical evaluations are indicated in Table 24-2.

Table 24-2
Results of Clinical Evaluations for Secondary Amenorrhea

	Serum FSH	Serum LH	Bleeding After Progesterone Challenge
Anorexia nervosa	Low	Low	No
Ovariectomy	High	High	No
Asherman syndrome	Normal	Normal	No

FSH = follicle-stimulating hormone; *LH* = luteinizing hormone.

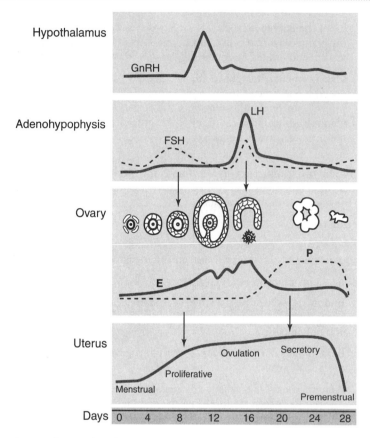

Figure 24-1. Hormonal control of the menstrual cycle. The hypothalamus secretes gonadotropin-releasing hormone (*GnRH*). In response to GnRH, the adenohypophysis secretes follicle-stimulating hormone (*FSH*) and luteinizing hormone (*LH*). In response to FSH, the development of a secondary follicle to a Graafian follicle is stimulated in the ovary. The granulosa cells within the secondary follicle and Graafian follicle secrete estrogen (*E*). In response to estrogen, the endometrium of the uterus enters the proliferative phase. In response to LH (LH surge), ovulation occurs. After ovulation, the granulosa lutein cells of the corpus luteum secrete progesterone (*P*). In response to progesterone, the endometrium of the uterus enters the secretory phase. Conditions that impair the secretion of GnRH from the hypothalamus will prevent the secretion of FSH that is necessary for follicle development and will result in infertility. In such cases, the drug **clomiphene** (an estrogen receptor antagonist) is used to increase GnRH secretion. In patients with **polycystic ovary syndrome,** increased LH secretion from the adenohypophysis stimulates excessive production of androgens by the theca interna cells of secondary and Graafian follicles, resulting in numerous atretic or cystic follicles.

4. **Menorrhagia** is excessive bleeding at menstruation in either the amount of blood or number of days. It is usually associated with a **leiomyoma.**

5. **Dysmenorrhea** is excessive pain during menstruation. It is commonly associated with **endometriosis** and an increased level of **prostaglandin F** in the menstrual fluid.

6. **Metrorrhagia** is bleeding that occurs at irregular intervals. It is commonly associated with **cervical carcinoma** or **cervical polyps.**

7. **Prepubertal bleeding** is bleeding that occurs before menarche. It is commonly associated with vaginitis, infection, sexual abuse, or embryonal rhabdomyosarcoma.

8. **Postmenopausal bleeding** occurs approximately 1 year after the cessation of the menstrual cycle. It is commonly associated with malignant tumors of the uterus.

V. CERVIX

A. During prepuberty, the **ectocervix** protrudes into the vagina and is covered by a **nonkeratinized, stratified squamous epithelium** that is continuous with the vaginal epithelium.

B. The **endocervical canal** connects the uterine cavity with the vaginal cavity and is lined by deep crypts of **mucous-secreting simple columnar epithelium.**

1. At puberty, the simple columnar epithelium of the endocervical canal extends onto the ectocervix. However, exposure of the simple columnar epithelium to the acidic (pH = 3) environment of the vagina induces a **squamous metaplasia** and the formation of a **transformation zone.**

2. The transformation zone is the site of **Nabothian cysts,** which develop as stratified squamous epithelium grows over the mucous-secreting simple columnar epithelium and entraps large amounts of mucus.

   a. The transformation zone is the most common site of **squamous cell carcinoma of the cervix,** which is usually preceded by epithelial changes called **cervical intraepithelial neoplasia,** which can be diagnosed by a Papanicolaou (Pap) smear.

   b. The **Pap smear** also may be used to evaluate hormonally a woman in many different clinical situations by establishing a **maturation index** based on the morphology of 100 cells (Table 24-3).

   (1) **Superficial squamous cells** form under the influence of estrogen.

   (2) **Intermediate squamous cells** form under the influence of progesterone.

   (3) **Parabasal cells** imply the absence of estrogen or progesterone influence.

VI. VAGINA is lined by nonkeratinized stratified squamous epithelium.

A. The **superficial cells** are continuously exfoliated during the menstrual cycle, but exfoliation increases during the late secretory phase and menstrual phase.

B. The **exfoliated cells** contain **glycogen,** which is metabolized by commensal lactobacilli to lactic acid, which forms an acidic (pH = 3) environment. The acidic environment deters the invasion of bacterial pathogens and fungi (e.g., *Candida albicans,* which causes vaginal thrush).

C. The labia major and clitoris may be sites of metastasis of a malignant melanoma.

D. *Trichomonas vaginalis* is a flagellated protozoan that is sexually transmitted. It produces a vaginitis characterized by an inflammatory Pap smear with numerous neutrophils, strawberry-colored mucosa, and discharge (leukorrhea). Postcoital bleeding is a common complaint. In a wet preparation of the vaginal discharge, the tumbling motility of the organism can be observed.

Table 24-3
Maturation Indices in Various Clinical Situations

	ISC	PBC	SSC
Normal nonpregnant adult woman	30	0	70
Estrogen tumor or therapy; polycystic ovarian syndrome	0	0	100
Pregnant woman; prepubescent girl	100	0	0
Menopausal woman	0	100	0

ISC = intermediate squamous cells; *PBC* = parabasal cells; *SSC* = superficial squamous cells.

E. *Gardnerella vaginalis* is a bacterial infection often associated with *Mobiluncus* or *Bacteroides*. It is not sexually transmitted. It produces a vaginitis characterized by no inflammatory Pap smear, no changes in the mucosa, and discharge. In the "sniff test" of the vaginal discharge, a drop of potassium hydroxide produces a noticeable fishy, amine-like smell.

VII. MAMMARY GLAND

A. At puberty

    1. The mammary gland consists of elongated **lactiferous ducts** and **solid masses of epithelial cells,** which are surrounded by **myoepithelial cells.**

    2. It accumulates adipose tissue, which is largely responsible for variations in breast size.

B. During pregnancy

    1. The mammary gland consists of rapidly growing **lactiferous ducts** and proliferating epithelial cells, which form **alveoli** due to increased levels of estrogen and progesterone from the ovary and placenta. Ducts and alveoli distend as alveoli secrete **colostrum** [protein-rich (e.g., antibodies) and lipid-poor].

    2. The gland loses adipose tissue.

C. After childbirth

    1. The mammary gland is stimulated by **prolactin** from the adenohypophysis so that the alveolar cells continuously secrete **milk** (protein-rich and lipid-rich) into the lumen of the alveoli.

    2. At feeding time, a **surge of prolactin** increases milk secretion, and a **surge of oxytocin** causes expulsion of accumulated milk (letdown reflex) by stimulating contraction of myoepithelial cells.

VIII. SELECTED PHOTOMICROGRAPHS

A. Proliferative and secretory phases of the endometrium (Figure 24-2; see IV A)

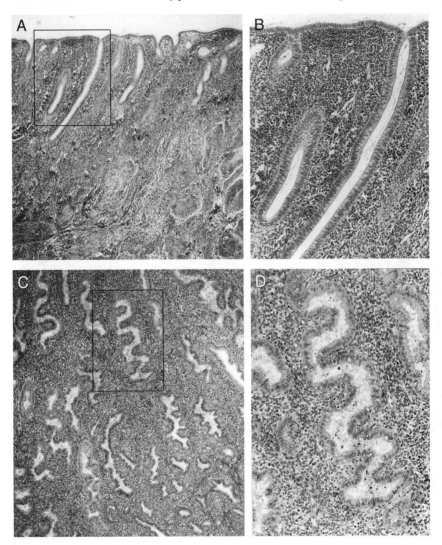

Figure 24-2. (A) Low magnification of the proliferative phase of the endometrium showing straight endometrial glands. (B) High magnification of the *boxed area in* A. (C) Low magnification of the secretory phase of the endometrium showing convoluted endometrium glands with secretion product within the lumen. (D) High magnification of the *boxed area in* C.

B. Cervix–vagina junction, cervical intraepithelial neoplasia, Pap smear (Figure 24-3; see V B 2)

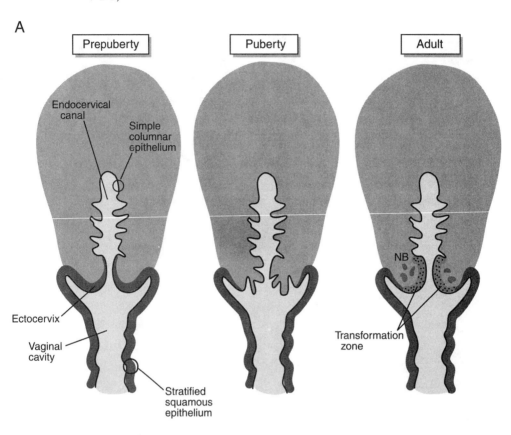

A

Prepuberty

Puberty

Adult

Endocervical canal

Simple columnar epithelium

NB

Ectocervix

Vaginal cavity

Transformation zone

Stratified squamous epithelium

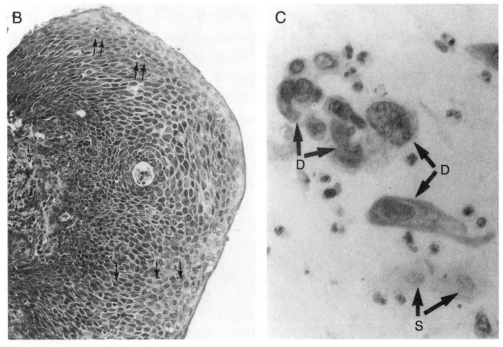

C. Squamous cell carcinoma of cervix (Figure 24-4)

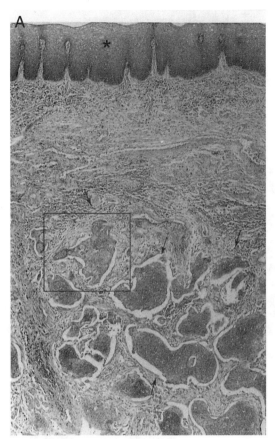
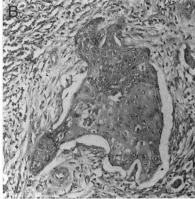

Figure 24-4. (*A,B*) Squamous cell carcinoma of the cervix. Cervical intraepithelial neoplasia, as explained in Figure 24-3, usually precedes the appearance of squamous cell carcinoma. Stratified squamous epithelium (*asterisk*) in the transformation zone has invaded the underlying stroma, forming nests of malignant cells (*arrows*). (*B*) High magnification of the *boxed area in A.* Squamous cell carcinoma can be treated clinically by radiation and chemotherapy with **cisplatin** or **5-fluorouracil.** (Reprinted with permission from East Carolina University, School of Medicine, Department of Pathology slide collection.)

Figure 24-3. (*A*) Diagram of the cervix–vaginal junction. During prepuberty, the ectocervix is covered by nonkeratinized stratified squamous epithelium that is continuous with vaginal epithelium (*black area*). At puberty, the simple columnar epithelium extends onto the ectocervix. In the adult, exposure of the simple columnar epithelium to the acidic (pH) environment of the vagina induces a squamous metaplasia, forming the transformation zone (*dotted area*), which is important clinically. Nabothian cysts (*NB*) may form in the transformation zone. (*B*) A biopsy of the cervix showing cervical intraepithelial neoplasia (*CIN*). In certain areas of the stratified squamous epithelium, the regular stratified pattern is lost such that cells near the surface are oriented vertically (*arrows*) instead of horizontally. There is a variation of nuclear size and shape. Mitotic figures near the surface can be observed (*double arrows*). (*C*) The cytology of cervical intraepithelial neoplasia as seen on a Pap smear. Normal cervical squamous cells (*S*) can be observed along with clumps of dysplastic cells (*D*), which have a large, darkly stained nuclei with a coarse chromatin pattern. (*B:* Reprinted with permission from East Carolina University, School of Medicine, Department of Pathology slide collection. *C:* Reprinted with permission from Wheater PR, Burkitt HG, Stevens A, et al: Identification of molecules in the kidney utilizing immunocytochemistry. In *Basic Histopathology: A Colour Atlas and Text*, 2nd ed. London, Churchill Livingstone, p 176, 1996, by permission of the publisher Churchill Livingstone.)

   D. Normal lactating breast, fibroadenoma (Figure 24-5; see VII C)

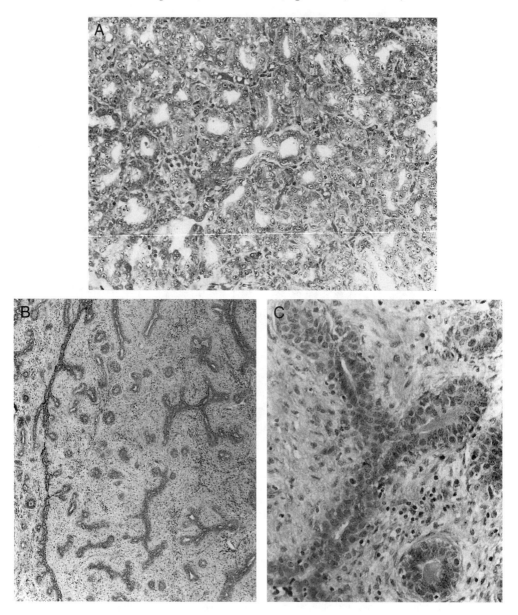

Figure 24-5. (A) Light micrograph of a normal, lactating breast. Observe the numerous round or oval alveoli surrounded by minimal connective tissue stroma. (B) Light micrograph of a fibroadenoma, which is a benign proliferation of the connective tissue stroma. As a consequence, the glands are compressed into cords of epithelium with slit-like spaces. (C) High magnification of a fibroadenoma showing glandular and stromal elements. A fibroadenoma presents clinically as a sharply circumscribed, spherical nodule that is freely movable. Reprinted with permission from East Carolina University, School of Medicine, Department of Pathology slide collection.

E. Infiltrating duct carcinoma of the breast (Figure 24-6)

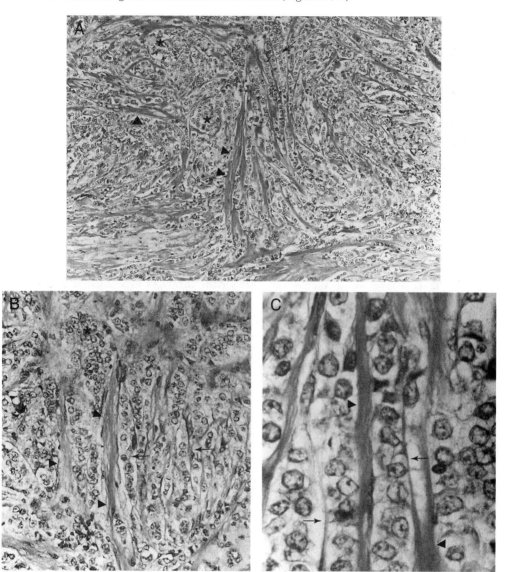

Figure 24-6. (A,B,C) Light micrographs of infiltrating duct carcinoma of the breast. The tumor cells are arranged in cell nests (*asterisk*), cell cords (*arrows*), anastomosing masses, or a mixture of all of these. The cells are surrounded by fairly thick bands of connective tissue stroma (*arrowheads*). This is the most common type of breast cancer, accounting for 65%–80% of all breast cancers. Some features that are common to all infiltrative breast carcinomas include: fixed in position, retraction and dimpling of the skin, thickening of the skin (peau d'orange), and retraction of the nipple. The presence of **estrogen receptors** or **progesterone receptors** within the carcinoma cells indicates a good prognosis for treatment. **Tamoxifen** is an estrogen receptor blocker and is a drug of choice for treatment. The presence of the **c-erb B2 oncoprotein** (similar to the epidermal growth factor receptor) on the surface of the carcinoma cells indicates a poor prognosis for treatment. **BRCA-1** (breast cancer susceptibility gene) is an anti-oncogene (tumor suppressor gene) located on chromosome 17 (17q21) that encodes for BRCA protein (a zinc finger gene-regulatory protein) containing phosphotyrosine, which will suppress the cell cycle. A mutation of the BRCA-1 gene is present in 5%–10% of women with breast cancer and confers a very high lifetime risk of breast and ovarian cancer.

25
Male Reproductive System

I. SEMINIFEROUS TUBULES of the testes are lined by two types of cells.

   A. Sertoli cells. These cells have the following functions.

      1. Sertoli cells provide mechanical and nutritional support for developing germ cells.

      2. They phagocytose excess cytoplasm discarded by spermatids.

      3. They form the **blood–testes barrier** through **tight junctions** on their lateral borders.

      4. These cells secrete **inhibin,** which inhibits release of follicle-stimulating hormone (FSH) from the adenohypophysis.

      5. They secrete **Müllerian inhibitory factor (MIF)** during fetal development, which inhibits development of the paramesonephric duct in a genotypic XY fetus.

      6. Sertoli cells synthesize **androgen-binding protein (ABP),** which binds testosterone so that high levels of testosterone are present in the seminiferous tubules, which is necessary for spermatogenesis to occur.

      7. They possess **FSH receptors** so that FSH from the adenohypophysis stimulates spermatogenesis and synthesis of ABP.

   B. Spermatogenic cells. The transformation of type A spermatogonia to sperm (called **spermatogenesis**) is described in three stages: **spermatocytogenesis, meiosis,** and **spermiogenesis** (Table 25-1).

II. SPERMIOGENESIS is a postmeiotic series of morphologic changes by which spermatids are transformed into sperm.

   A. Golgi phase. Numerous **proacrosomal granules** appear in the Golgi complex and coalesce to form one large granule within the **acrosomal vesicle.**

   B. Cap phase. The acrosomal vesicle covers the nucleus.

   C. Acrosome phase

      1. The large acrosome granule diffuses throughout the acrosomal vesicle, thereby forming the **acrosome.**

      2. The nuclear chromatin condenses into a dense mass.

      3. An array of microtubules called the **manchette** assists in the elongation of the spermatid.

      4. Centrioles migrate to the posterior pole of the spermatid and initiate the formation of the **axoneme (cilium)** of the sperm tail.

Table 25-1
Stages of Spermatogenesis

	Cell Type	(Number of Chromosomes, Amount of DNA)	Description
Spermiogenesis	Sperm	(23,1N)	Newly formed sperm are immotile Develop **motility** within the epididymis Undergo **capacitation** in the female reproductive tract before fertilization is possible
	Spermatids	(23,1N)	Undergo spermiogenesis to form sperm
Meiosis	Secondary spermatocytes	(23,2N)	Complete meiosis II within a **few hours** to form 4 spermatids
	Primary spermatocytes	(46,4N)	Remain in prophase for **22 days,** during which changing nuclear chromatin patterns can be described: **lepototene** (long, thin DNA strands), **zygotene** (synapsis occurs), **pachytene** (short, thick coiled DNA), and **diplotene** (chromosomes separate except at centromere) Complete meiosis I to form 2 secondary spermatocytes
Spermatocyto-genesis	Type B spermatogonia	(46,2N)	Enter meiosis I and undergo DNA replication to form primary spermatocytes
	Type A spermatogonia	(46,2N)	Undergo mitosis to form either more type A spermatogonia (to maintain the supply) or type B spermatogonia

5. A mitochondrial sheath forms around the axoneme.

6. Outer dense fibers and a fibrous sheath form around the axoneme.

D. Maturation phase

    1. Excess spermatid cytoplasm is discarded and phagocytosed by Sertoli cells.

    2. Intercellular bridges are lost.

III. SPERM MORPHOLOGY (Figure 25-1)

IV. LEYDIG (INTERSTITIAL) CELLS are found in connective tissue between the seminiferous tubules. They contain **crystals of Reinke** within the cytoplasm.

A. Functions

    1. Leydig cells possess **LH receptors** so that LH from the adenohypophysis stimulates testosterone secretion.

    2. Leydig cells secrete **testosterone.**

        a. Testosterone gives rise to two other potent androgens:

            (1) **Dihydrotestosterone (DHT)** is produced from testosterone via the enzyme **5α-reductase.**

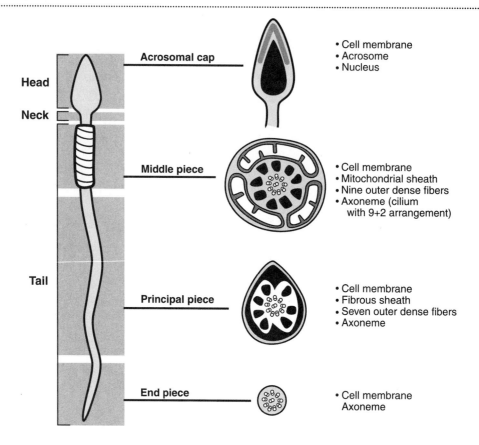

Left-side labels: Head, Neck, Tail

Right-side section labels and composition:

Acrosomal cap
- Cell membrane
- Acrosome
- Nucleus

Middle piece
- Cell membrane
- Mitochondrial sheath
- Nine outer dense fibers
- Axoneme (cilium with 9+2 arrangement)

Principal piece
- Cell membrane
- Fibrous sheath
- Seven outer dense fibers
- Axoneme

End piece
- Cell membrane
  Axoneme

Figure 25-1.   Diagram of human sperm. Regions of the mature sperm are shown on the *left*. Sections through the head, middle piece, principal piece, and end piece along with their composition are shown on the *right*.

   (2) **5α-Androstanediol** is produced from testosterone via the enzyme **3α-reductase.**

b. Aromatization of testosterone and androstenedione within the liver and adipose tissue by P_{450} **aromatase** produces significant amounts of estradiol and estrone in males.

c. During **fetal life,** testosterone is essential in the development of the epididymis, ductus deferens, seminal vesicle, and ejaculatory duct to produce the male phenotype in a genotypic XY fetus. DHT is essential for the development of the penis and scrotum (external genitalia) and prostate gland.

d. During **puberty and adult life,** androgens are essential for spermatogenesis; function of prostate, seminal vesicle, and bulbourethral glands; appearance of secondary sex characteristics; closure of the epiphyseal growth plate; increase in muscle mass; and lipid metabolism [testosterone increases low-density lipoprotein (LDL) and decreases high-density lipoprotein (HDL)].

e. Between 1% and 2% of circulating testosterone is in the free form; the remainder is bound to a liver-derived **sex steroid-binding globulin** or **albumin.**

f. Plasma testosterone levels during the lifespan of a normal male are shown in Figure 25-2.

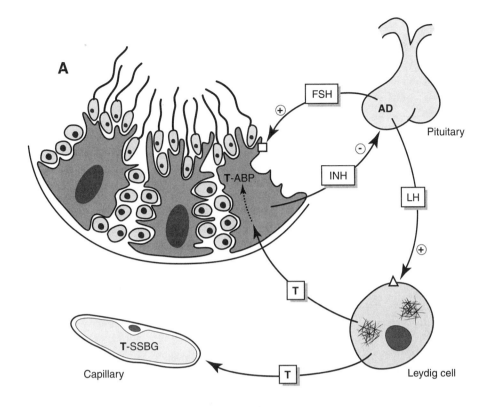

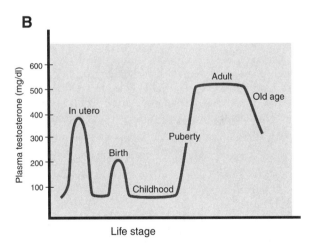

Figure 25-2. (A) Diagram of hormonal control of the male reproductive system. The adenohypophysis (*AD*) secretes follicle-stimulating hormone (*FSH*) and luteinizing hormone (*LH*). FSH binds to FSH receptors (*box*) on the Sertoli cells (*shaded*), which stimulates the synthesis of androgen-binding protein (*ABP*). The Sertoli cells secrete inhibin (*INH*), which inhibits FSH secretion (a feedback loop). LH binds to LH receptors (*triangle*) on the Leydig cells, which stimulates the secretion of testosterone (*T*). Testosterone circulates in the blood bound to sex steroid-binding globulin (SSBG). Testosterone binds to ABP within Sertoli cells to maintain high levels of testosterone necessary for spermatogenesis. (*B*) Plasma testosterone levels during the lifespan of a normal male. The peak testosterone levels during in utero development (0–9months) produce the male phenotype in a genotypic XY fetus. The physiologic significance of the peak at birth is not known. Plasma testosterone levels increase steeply at puberty, plateau in the adult at approximately 600 ng/dl, and begin to decline in old age. (Based on data from Griffin JE et al: The testes. In *Metabolic Control and Disease*. Edited by Bondy PK, Rosenberg LE. Philadelphia, Saunders, 1980; and Winter JSD, Hughes IA, Reyes FI, et al: Pituitary–gonadal relations in infancy. *J Clin Endocrinol Metabol* l42: 679, 1976.)

V. PROSTATE GLAND

A. Anatomy. The prostate gland is a collection of tubuloalveolar glands arranged in three concentric groups (mucosal, submucosal, and main), all of which empty into the urethra. The lumen of the tubuloalveolar glands contain deposits known as **corpus amylacea.**

B. Functions

   1. The prostate gland secretes acid phosphatase, fibrinolysin, citric acid, amylase, and prostate-specific antigen (PSA). **Serum levels of acid phosphatase and PSA** are used in the diagnosis and management of prostate cancer.

   2. DHT is the main mediator of prostatic growth. This is clinically important in benign prostatic hypertrophy because **finasteride** (a 5α-reductase inhibitor) can reduce DHT levels and shrink the size of the prostate gland. In addition, the action of DHT can be blocked by the receptor antagonist called **flutamide.**

VI. CLINICAL CONSIDERATIONS

A. Complete androgen insensitivity (CAIS; testicular feminization syndrome) is caused by a mutation in the **androgen receptor (AR) gene** that renders the AR inactive. It is the most common cause of male pseudointersexuality.

   1. Normally, the AR is a **nuclear transcription factor** that is activated by androgens to bind DNA promoter regions that regulate transcription of other genes.

   2. CAIS produces the following clinical findings: 46,XY genotype and undescended testes, but normal-appearing female external genitalia; uterus and uterine tubes are absent.

   3. These individuals present as normal-appearing females, and their psychosocial orientation is female despite their genotype.

B. 5α-Reductase 2 deficiency is caused by a mutation in the **5α-reductase 2 gene** that renders the 5α-reductase 2 enzyme inactive.

   1. Normally, 5α-reductase 2 catalyzes the conversion of testosterone to DHT.

   2. It produces the following clinical findings: underdevelopment of the penis, scrotum (microphallus, hypospadias, and bifid scrotum), and prostate gland. The epididymis, ductus deferens, seminal vesicle, and ejaculatory duct are normal. These clinical findings have led to inference that DHT is essential for the development of the external genitalia and prostate gland in genotypic XY fetuses.

   3. At puberty, these individuals demonstrate a striking virilization.

   4. An increased **testosterone:DHT ratio** is diagnostic (normal = 5; 5α-reductase 2 deficiency = 20–60).

C. 17α-Hydroxysteroid dehydrogenase 3 (HSD) deficiency is caused by a mutation in the **17α-HSD 3 gene** that renders the 17α-HSD 3 enzyme inactive. It is the most common defect in androgen biosynthesis.

   1. Normally, 17α-HSD 3 catalyzes the conversion of androstenedione to testosterone.

   2. It produces the following clinical findings: underdevelopment of the penis and scrotum (microphallus, hypospadias, and bifid scrotum) and prostate gland. The epididymis, ductus deferens, seminal vesicle, and ejaculatory duct are normal. The clinical findings in 17α-HSD deficiency and 5α-reductase 2 deficiency are very similar.

D. Testicular lymphoma is a metastatic malignant lymphoma that presents as a testicular mass. It is the most common form of testicular cancer in men older than 60 years.

E. Yolk sac tumor (endodermal sinus tumor) is the most common form of testicular cancer in infants and children up to 3 years of age. It secretes α-fetoprotein, which is used a tumor marker.

VII. SELECTED PHOTOMICROGRAPHS

A. Seminiferous tubule (Figure 25-3; see I)

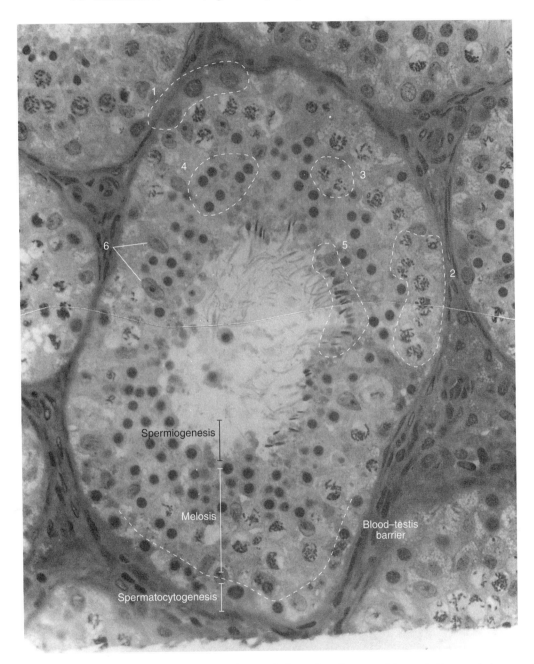

Figure 25-3.   Light micrograph of seminiferous tubules within the testes. The seminiferous tubules contain spermatogonia (*1*), primary spermatocytes (*2*) , secondary spermatocytes (*3*), early spermatids (*4*), late spermatids (*5*), and Sertoli cells (*6*). In addition, the three stages of spermatogenesis (i.e., spermatocytogenesis, meiosis, and spermiogenesis) are indicated by the *brackets* (correlate with Table 25-1). The level of the blood–testis barrier is indicated by the *dotted line*.

B. Leydig cells (Figure 25-4; see IV)

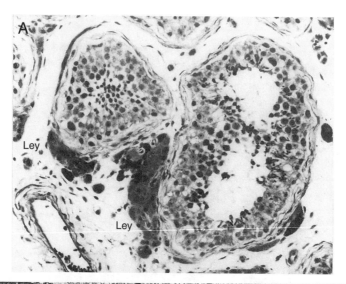

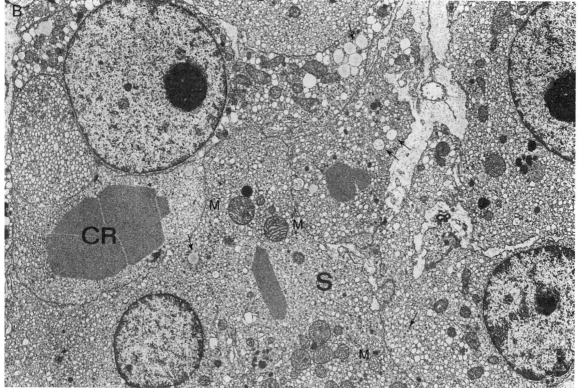

Figure 25-4. (A) Light micrograph of Leydig cells (*Ley*) found in the connective tissue between the seminiferous tubules. (B) Electron micrograph of Leydig cells. Smooth endoplasmic reticulum (S), mitochondria with tubular cristae (M), and lipid droplets (*arrows*) are typically found in a steroid-secreting cell. CR = crystals of Reinke. (Reprinted with permission from Kerr JB: Ultrastructure of the seminiferous epithelium and intertubular tissue of the human testis. *J Electron Microsc Tech* 19(2): 215–240, 1991. © 1991 Wiley-Liss. Reprinted by permission of Wiley-Liss, Inc., a subsidiary of John Wiley & Sons, Inc.)

C. Seminoma (Figure 25-5)

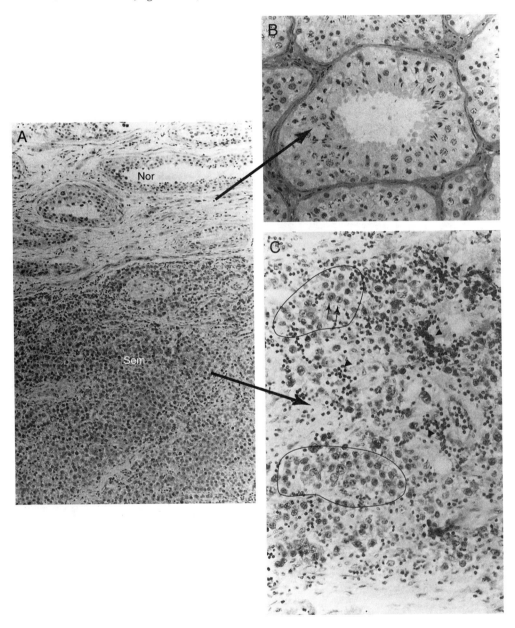

Figure 25-5.   Light micrograph of seminoma. Approximately 95% of testicular neoplasms arise from germ cells. Almost all germ cell neoplasms involve the isochromosome of the short arm of chromosome 12 [i(12p)], which is virtually diagnostic. Seminoma is the most common type of germ cell neoplasm. (A) Low-power light micrograph of a seminoma showing normal testicular tissue at the periphery (*Nor*) with typical seminiferous tubules and seminoma (*Sem*). (B) High magnification showing normal testicular tissue at the periphery with typical seminiferous tubules. (C) High magnification of a seminoma, which consists of clusters of moderately sized round cells with large centrally located nuclei with prominent nucleoli (*outlined areas*). Mitotic figures can be observed (*arrows*). The cell clusters are separated by fibrous cords (*arrowheads in A*). The fibrous cords are heavily infiltrated with lymphocytes (*arrowheads in C*), which may play a role in the immune rejection of seminomas and contribute to the favorable prognosis of these neoplasms. (Reprinted with permission from East Carolina University, School of Medicine, Department of Pathology slide collection.)

D. Testicular teratocarcinoma (Figure 25-6)

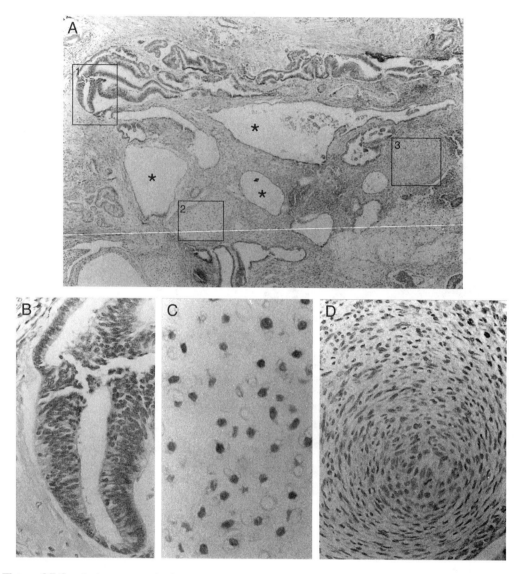

Figure 25-6.   Light micrograph of testicular teratocarcinoma (*TC*). Teratocarcinoma is another type of germ-cell neoplasm that is composed of a collection of well-differentiated cells or structures from each of the three primary germ layers. (A) Teratocarcinoma is composed of a fibrous stroma with many cyst-like structures (*asterisk*). In addition, well-differentiated glandular structures resembling colon glandular epithelium (endoderm; *box 1*), cartilage (mesoderm; *box 2*), and squamous epithelium (ectoderm; *box 3*). (B) High magnification of glandular structures. (C) High magnification of cartilage. (D) High magnification of squamous epithelium. (Reprinted with permission from East Carolina University, School of Medicine, Department of Pathology slide collection.)

E. Normal prostate gland (Figure 25-7; see V)

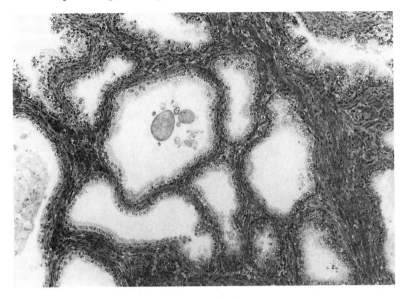

Figure 25-7.   Light micrograph of normal prostate gland. Tubuloalveolar glands are lined by a simple columnar epithelium surrounded by a connective tissue stroma. Corpus amylacea are observed within the lumen.

F. Benign prostatic hyperplasia (Figure 25-8)

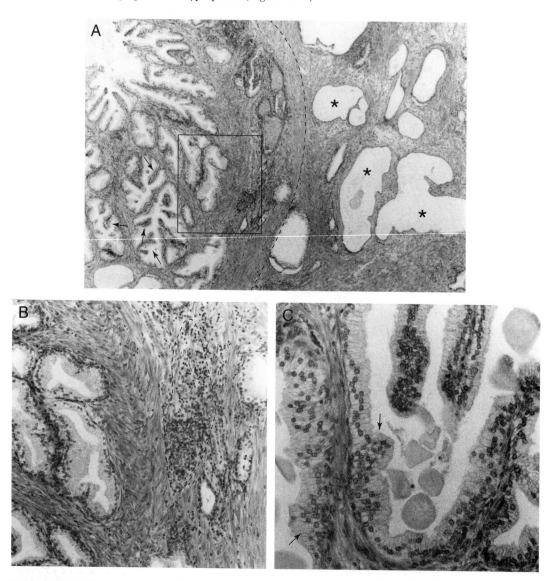

Figure 25-8.   Light micrograph of benign prostatic hyperplasia, which is the most common disorder of the prostate gland and generally occurs in elderly men. The **mucosal and submucosal glands** close to the urethra are characteristically enlarged so that compression of the urethra occurs with resulting **difficulty in urination.** Dihydrotestosterone is the main mediator of prostate growth. In older men, 17β-estradiol levels increase and may sensitize the prostate gland to the effects of dihydrotestosterone. (A) Low magnification shows a proliferation of both glands within a fairly well-defined nodule (*dotted lines*) and the connective tissue stroma. The epithelium of the glands characteristically forms papillary buds or infoldings (*arrows*), which are much more prominent than in the normal prostate. Other glands are cystically dilated (*asterisk*). (B) High magnification of the *boxed area in A* shows hyperplastic glands and stroma infiltrated by lymphocytes (*dotted area*). (C) High-magnification hyperplastic glands lined by a conspicuous epithelium of tall columnar cells that appear multilayered in some locations (*arrows*). Within the lumen, corpus amylacea and papillary buds or infoldings can be seen. (Reprinted with permission from East Carolina University, School of Medicine, Department of Pathology slide collection.)

G. Prostatic carcinoma (Figure 25-9)

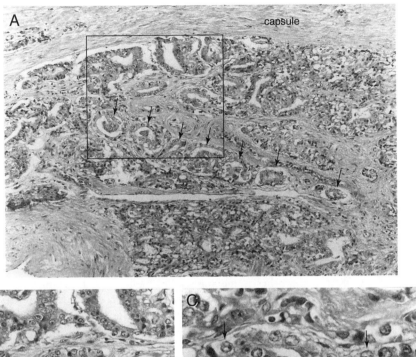

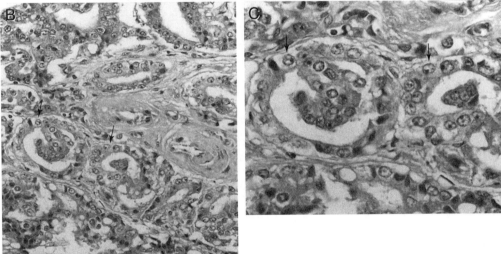

Figure 25-9.   Light micrograph of prostatic carcinoma (PC). PC is the most common form of cancer in men. PC generally starts in the **main glands of the prostate** located at the periphery near the capsule. Therefore, by the time blockage of the urethra occurs, PC is already in an advanced state. The most reliable sign of malignancy is the invasion of the capsule that contains lymphatics, blood vessels, and nerves. The finding of osteoblastic metastasis in bone, particularly lumbar vertebral bodies, is diagnostic of PC. (A) Low magnification of PC showing the main glands of the prostate near the capsule. Numerous small malignant acini can be observed lying side-by-side to each other (*arrows*). (B, C) High magnification of the *boxed area in* A shows malignant acini lined by cuboidal epithelium (*arrows*). The acini may be filled with cell nests. In a poorly differentiated PC, acini are not apparent; instead, cords of neoplastic cells invade the stroma. (Reprinted with permission from East Carolina University, School of Medicine, Department of Pathology slide collection.)

26
Skin

I. EPIDERMIS. This layer is classified as stratified squamous epithelium.

   A. **Keratinocytes** are arranged in five strata: **corneum, lucidum, granulosum, spinosum,** and **basale** (Table 26-1).

   B. Nonkeratinocytes

   1. **Melanocytes** are found in **stratum basale.**
      a. They synthesize **melanin** in organelles called **melanosomes.** Melanosomes contain **tyrosinase,** which catalyzes the conversion of tyrosine to dihydroxyphenylalanine (DOPA) to melanin.
      b. They transfer melanin to neighboring keratinocytes via cell processes that contain melanosomes.

   2. **Merkel cells** are found in **stratum basale.**
      a. They contain many **dense-core granules.**
      b. They are associated with sensory nerve endings and function as **mechano-receptors.**

   3. **Langerhans cells** are found in **stratum spinosum.**
      a. They contain **Birbeck granules.**
      b. These **antigen-presenting cells** originate in the bone marrow and participate in type IV delayed-type reactions (see Chapter 9 VI D).

II. DERMIS is composed of type I collagen and elastic fibers.

III. GLANDS

   A. **Eccrine sweat glands** have the following characteristics:
   1. Eccrine sweat glands secrete a watery product (composed of sodium, chloride, potassium, urea, and ammonia) via merocrine secretion.
   2. They open onto the skin surface as sweat pores.
   3. They are widely distributed throughout the body.
   4. They are active throughout life.
   5. These glands regulate body temperature via postganglionic sympathetic neurons that use acetylcholine (cholinergic) (Note: As a rule, postganglionic sympathetic neurons use norepinephrine as their neurotransmitter; however, there is an exception to the rule in the regulation of body temperature).
   6. Eccrine sweat glands regulate emotional sweating via postganglionic sympathetic neurons that use norepinephrine (adrenergic).

Table 26-1
Characteristics of Keratinocytes

Strata	Characteristics
Stratum corneum	Nucleus and organelles absent Thickened cell membrane due to deposition of a protein called **involucrin** Cytoplasm filled with keratin intermediate filaments surrounded by a matrix derived from filaggrin
Stratum lucidum	Nucleus absent A highly refractive transitional zone Quite apparent only in thick skin of palms and soles
Stratum granulosum	Contains keratohyaline granules Contains lamellar bodies, which begin to secrete an impermeable water barrier Contains keratin intermediate filaments Contains a protein associated with keratin called **filaggrin**
Stratum spinosum	Numerous desmosomes Contains keratin intermediate filaments Contains lamellar bodies
Stratum basale	Attached to basement membrane via hemidesmosomes Contains keratin intermediate filaments Mitotically active

B. **Apocrine sweat glands** have the following characteristics:

  1. Apocrine sweat glands secrete a viscous product via merocrine secretion.

  2. They open into the pilosebaceous canal of a hair shaft.

  3. They are under endocrine control (androgens and estrogens).

  4. These glands are found in the axilla, mons pubis, and anal regions.

  5. They are active at puberty and play a role in malodorous body scent.

  6. Apocrine sweat glands produce pheromones ("sexual attraction") via postganglionic sympathetic neurons that use norepinephrine (adrenergic).

C. **Sebaceous glands** have the following characteristics:

  1. Sebaceous glands secrete sebum (composed of triglycerides, wax esters, squalene, and cholesterol) via holocrine secretion.

  2. They open into the pilosebaceous canal of a hair shaft.

  3. They are under endocrine control; androgens increase activity, whereas estrogens decrease activity.

  4. Sebaceous glands are active at puberty and may play a role in **acne.**

IV. NERVES

  A. **Motor nerves** activate glands and control blood flow.

  B. **Sensory nerves**

  1. Free nerve endings
  a. Myelinated axons lose their myelin sheath, enter the epidermis, and terminate in the stratum granulosum.

    b. They may function in pain and temperature sensation.

2. Merkel endings

    a. Myelinated axons end in disk-like expansions that terminate on Merkel cells in the stratum basale.

    b. They may function as a mechanoreceptor.

3. Meissner's corpuscles

    a. A myelinated axon enters a connective tissue capsule within the dermal papillae and pursues a zigzag course among modified Schwann cells.

    b. They may function as mechanoreceptors.

4. Pacinian corpuscles

    a. A myelinated axon in the dermis enters a connective tissue capsule within the dermis and hypodermis and loses its myelin sheath.

    b. The unmyelinated axon is surrounded by 20–60 concentric layers of cells and gelatinous material (onion appearance).

    c. They may function as a mechanoreceptor and a vibration receptor.

V. CLINICAL CONSIDERATIONS

A. **Malignant melanoma** is a skin lesion with irregular borders and striking variations in pigmentation. Melanomas involve the transformation of melanocytes from highly dendritic cells to oval cells that grow in nests. **Dysplastic nevi** are precursors of malignant melanoma.

B. **Vitiligo** is a disorder characterized by the loss of melanocytes, resulting in patches of hypopigmented skin most noticeable in darkly pigmented individuals. This disorder contrasts with **albinism,** in which melanocytes are present but lack the enzyme tyrosinase so that no melanin pigment is produced.

C. **Epidermolysis bullosa (EB)** is a group of hereditary diseases that affect the epidermal–dermal adhesion and result clinically in blistering. Mutations in the genes for keratin, laminin, integrin, bullous pemphigoid antigen (type XVII collagen), and type VII collagen have been implicated.

27

Ear

I. TYMPANIC MEMBRANE (EARDRUM) consists of three layers.

    A. Keratinized stratified squamous epithelium covers the external surface.

    B. Connective tissue that is vascularized and innervated constitutes the middle layer.

    C. Simple squamous epithelium covers the internal surface.

II. MEMBRANOUS LABYRINTH is contained within the osseous labyrinth. The membranous labyrinth is filled with endolymph. The osseous labyrinth is filled with perilymph.

    A. Kinetic labyrinth (semicircular ducts; Figure 27-1A)

        1. Type I and **type II hair cells** within **cristae ampullaris** have stereocilia and a single cilium (**kinocilium**) on their apical border. These cells are in contact with bipolar neurons of the vestibular ganglion of cranial nerve (CN) VIII.

        2. The kinetic labyrinth also contains supporting cells.

        3. Hair cells and supporting cells are covered by a gelatinous mass called a **cupula.**

        4. The semicircular ducts respond to **angular acceleration** and **deceleration of the head.**

    B. Static labyrinth (utricle and saccule; Figure 27-1B)

        1. Type I and **type II hair cells** within **maculae** have stereocilia and a single cilium (**kinocilium**) on their apical border. These cells are in contact with bipolar neurons of the vestibular ganglion of CN VIII.

        2. The static labyrinth also contains supporting cells.

        3. Hair cells and supporting cells are covered by a gelatinous mass called the **otolithic membrane,** which contains calcium carbonate crystals (**otoliths**).

        4. The utricle and saccule respond to the position of the head with respect to **linear acceleration** and **pull of gravity.**

    C. Cochlear duct (Figure 27-1C; Figure 27-2)

        1. This triangular duct comprises a **vestibular membrane** (roof), **basilar membrane** (floor), and **stria vascularis** (lateral wall). The stria vascularis participates in the formation of endolymph.

        2. The cochlear duct contains the **organ of Corti.**

            a. The organ of Corti contains **inner** and **outer hair cells** that have stereocilia (but no kinocilium) on their apical border and are in contact with bipolar neurons of the cochlear ganglion of CN VIII.

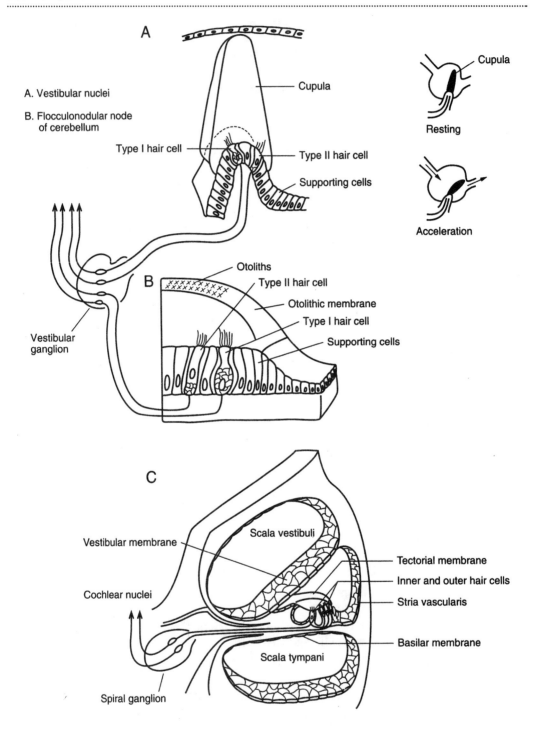

Figure 27-1. (A) Kinetic labyrinth (semicircular ducts). Note the deflection of the cupula during acceleration, which stimulates the hair cells. (B) Static labyrinth (utricle and saccule). (C) Cochlear duct. The organ of Corti is the receptor for sound. The scala vestibuli and scala tympani are part of the osseous labyrinth and are filled with perilymph.

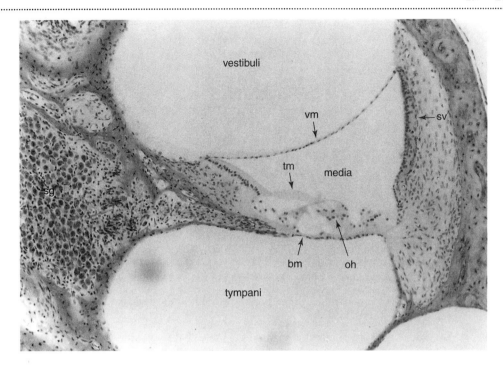

Figure 27-2. Light micrograph of the cochlear duct containing the organ of Corti. Note the vestibular membrane (*vm*), tectorial membrane (*tm*), basilar membrane (*bm*), bipolar neurons of the spiral ganglion (*sg*), stria vascularis (*sv*), outer hair cells (*oh*), scala vestibuli containing perilymph (*vestibuli*), scala media containing endolymph (*media*), and scala tympani containing perilymph (*tympani*).

    b. It also contains different types of supporting cells.
    c. Hair cells and supporting cells are covered by a gelatinous mass called the **tectorial membrane.**
    d. The organ of Corti responds to **sounds,** which induce vibrations of the basilar membrane.

III. CLINICAL CONSIDERATION. The organ of Corti may be damaged by exposure to rubella virus during week 7 and week 8 of embryologic development.

28
Eye

I. CORNEA

A. The central portion of this **avascular** structure receives nutrients via **diffusion from the aqueous humor** within the anterior chamber of the eye. The peripheral portion receives nutrients via diffusion from **blood vessels of the limbus.**

B. It is highly innervated by branches of the **ophthalmic division of the trigeminal nerve (cranial nerve [CN] V_1).**

C. The cornea is composed of five layers (Table 28-1).

II. LIMBUS

A. Located at the **sclerocorneal junction,** it contains a **trabecular network** and the **canal of Schlemm.**

B. The limbus is involved in the flow of aqueous humor: anterior chamber→trabecular network→canal of Schlemm→aqueous veins→episcleral veins.

C. Obstruction of flow of aqueous humor results in **glaucoma.**

III. RETINA. The 10 layers that constitute the retina are described and illustrated in Table 28-2 and Figure 28-1. The retina has a number of specialized areas, which include the following:

A. The **optic disk** is the site where optic nerve fibers converge to form the optic nerve (CN II). The optic disk lacks rods and cones and is therefore a blind spot.

B. **Macula** is a small yellow area (due to xanthophil pigment) located lateral to the optic disk. At the center of the macula is the **fovea,** which is composed exclusively of cones linked to a single ganglion cell, thereby producing the highest visual acuity and color vision.

IV. VISUAL TRANSDUCTION includes the following steps:

A. In the dark, rods have open sodium ion channels, which maintain the rod in a constant state of depolarization.

B. **Rhodopsin** is formed when **11-*cis*-retinal** binds to a glycoprotein called **opsin.** In light, 11-*cis*-retinal forms the isomer **all-*trans*-retinal,** which releases from opsin and is converted to **vitamin A** (retinol).

C. This activates a G protein called **transducin.**

D. Transducin activates cyclic guanosine monophosphate (cGMP) phosphodiesterase, which hydrolyzes cGMP to GMP, thereby **lowering cGMP levels.**

Table 28-1

Layers of the Cornea

Layers	Characteristics
Corneal epithelium	Anterior aspect of cornea (exposed to air) Stratified squamous epithelium (nonkeratinized) Many free nerve endings High capacity for regeneration
Bowman's membrane	A basement membrane
Stroma	Thickest layer of the cornea Collagen types III and V
Descemet's membrane	A basement membrane
Corneal endothelium	Posterior aspect of cornea (exposed to aqueous humor) Responsible for metabolic exchanges between cornea and aqueous humor Simple squamous epithelium

E. Low cGMP levels **close sodium ion channels, thereby eliciting a hyperpolarization.**

F. Visual transduction is quite different from the way action potentials in muscle and nerve are generated. In muscle and nerve, stimuli open sodium ion channels, thereby eliciting a depolarization (see Chapter 6 I G and Chapter 7 I B 4).

Table 28-2

Layers of the Retina

Layers	Characteristics
10 Inner limiting membrane	Termination of Muller cells and their basement membrane
9 Optic nerve fibers	Unmyelinated axons of ganglion cells
8 Ganglion cells	Nuclei of ganglion cells **Site of action potential generation**
7 Inner plexiform layer	Synapses between axons of bipolar cells and dendrites of ganglion cells
6 Inner nuclear layer	Nuclei of horizontal, bipolar, amacrine, and Muller cells
5 Outer plexiform layer	Synapses between axons of bipolar cells and dendrites of ganglion cells Retinal blood vessels may extend to this layer
4 Outer nuclear layer	Nuclei of rods and cones
3 Outer limiting membrane	Zonula adherens between rods/cones and Muller cells
2 Photoreceptor layer	Outer segment with membrane disks containing **Na$^+$ ion channels,** connecting cilium, and inner segment of rods and cones
	Detached retina occurs between 1 and 2
1 Pigment epithelium	Has tight junctions at apical border to form blood–retina barrier Has basal infoldings Contains melanin granules Esterifies retinol (vitamin A) Phagocytoses shed tips of rod outer segments

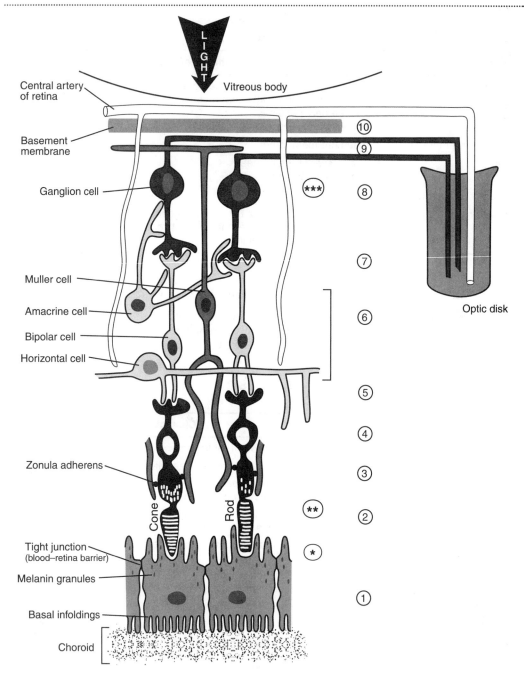

Figure 28-1.   Diagram of the retina. Tight junctions between the pigment epithelial cells establish a blood-retina barrier. Therefore, blood supply to the retina is from the central artery of the retina (a branch of the ophthalmic artery), not from vessels within the choroid. As retinal blood vessels leave the *optic disk,* they travel between the inner limiting membrane (*layer 10*) and the *vitreous body.* Retinal blood vessels may extend as far as the outer plexiform layer (*layer 5*) and play an important role in diabetic retinopathy. *Müller cells* act as supporting glial-type cells. Note the direction of the incident light and that it must pass through many layers of the retina before reaching the rods and cones. The *asterisk* indicates the site of retinal detachment; the *double asterisk* indicates the presence of sodium ion channels; the *triple asterisk* indicates the site of action potential generation.

V. CLINICAL CONSIDERATIONS

A. Retinitis pigmentosa is a genetic disease characterized by degeneration of rods, night blindness (nyctalopia), and "gun barrel" vision. Retinitis pigmentosa may be caused by abetalipoproteinemia (Bassen-Kornzweig syndrome) and may be arrested by massive doses of vitamin A.

B. Diabetic retinopathy. In patients with diabetes, retinal blood vessels frequently become leaky and exude fluid into the retina (particularly in the macula), leading to loss of visual acuity. It is the leading cause of blindness in the developed world and may be reduced by strict regulation of blood glucose levels.

C. Papilledema is edema of the optic disk (papilla) due to increased intracranial pressure usually caused by brain tumors, subdural hematoma, or hydrocephalus.

D. Night blindness (nyctalopia) is a condition in which vision in poor illumination is defective due to vitamin A (retinol) deficiency. An aldehyde of vitamin A (retinol) called retinal is the chromophore component of rhodopsin.

E. Retinoblastoma (Rb) is a tumor of the retina that occurs in childhood and develops from precursor cells in the immature retina.

  1. The **Rb gene** is located on chromosome 13 and encodes for Rb protein, which binds to a gene regulatory protein and causes suppression of the cell cycle [i.e., the Rb gene is a tumor-suppressor gene (also called an anti-oncogene)].

  2. A mutation in the Rb gene encodes an abnormal Rb protein such that there is **no suppression of the cell cycle.** This leads to the formation of retinoblastoma.
     a. **Hereditary retinoblastoma** causes multiple tumors in both eyes.
     b. **Nonhereditary retinoblastoma** causes one tumor in one eye.

VI. SELECTED PHOTOMICROGRAPHS

A. Cornea, retina, iris, and ciliary body (Figure 28-2)

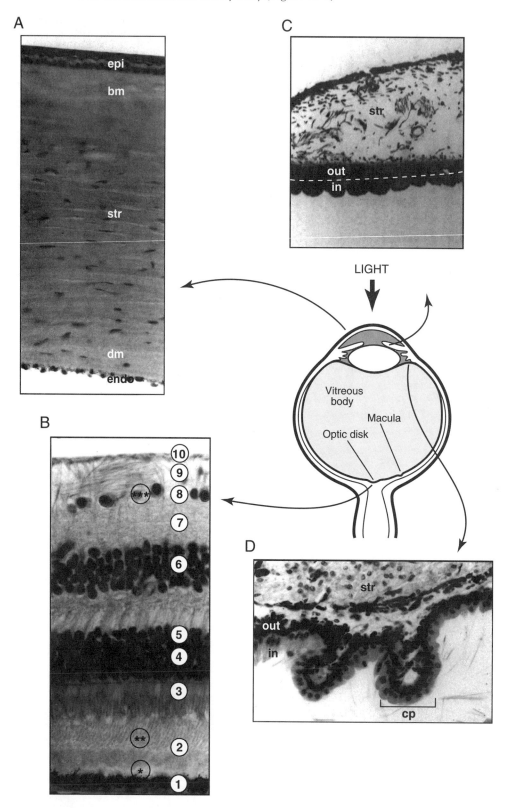

B. Rod outer segment (Figure 28-3)

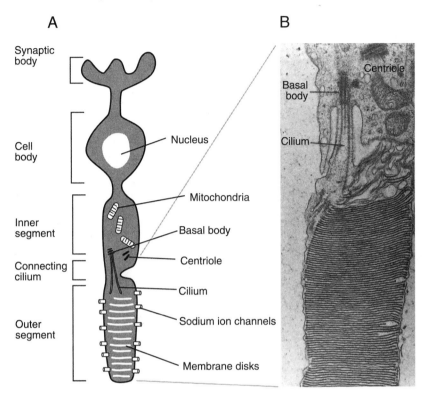

Figure 28-3. (A) Various portions of a rod. The outer segment has sodium ion channels on the cell membrane and contains membrane disks. The connecting cilium, inner segment, cell body, and synaptic body are also shown. (B) Electron micrograph of the outer segment (OS) and connecting cilium (CC). Note the cilium, basal body, and centriole. (B Reprinted with permission from Fawcett DW: A Textbook of Histology, 12th ed. New York, Chapman Hall, 1994, p 902. Courtesy of T. Kuwabara.)

Figure 28-2. (A) Light micrograph of cornea. The five layers of the cornea are indicated. *epi* = corneal epithelium; *bm* = Bowman's membrane; *str* = stroma; *dm* = Descemet's membrane; *endo* = corneal endothelium. (B) Light micrograph of retina. The 10 layers of the retina are indicated. The *asterisk* indicates the site of retinal detachment; the *double asterisk* indicates the presence of sodium ion channels; the *triple asterisk* indicates the site of action potential generation. (C) Light micrograph of iris. The posterior surface of the iris is lined by two layers of simple columnar epithelium, which are derived embryologically from the outer pigment layer (*out*) and inner (*in*) neural layer of the optic cup. Both of these layers are so highly pigmented that the two cell layers cannot be distinguished (see *dotted line* for boundary). The iris contains the dilator pupillae muscle and sphincter pupillae muscle, which are formed from the epithelium of the outer pigment layer (*out*) by a transformation of these epithelial cells into contractile cells. The stroma (*str*) of the iris contains connective tissue, blood vessels, nerves, and melanocytes. The number of melanocytes in the stroma determines eye color. (D) Light micrograph of ciliary body. The ciliary body is lined by two layers of simple columnar epithelium, which are derived embryologically from the outer pigment layer (*out*) and inner neural layer (*in*) of the optic cup. The outer pigment layer is pigmented, but the inner neural layer is nonpigmented. The ciliary body is thrown into folds called ciliary processes (*cp*). Both layers of epithelium are involved in the production of aqueous humor and suspensory fibers of the lens. The stroma (*str*) of the ciliary body contains connective tissue and the ciliary muscle.

29

Cerebral Cortex

I. CYTOARCHITECTURE. The neurons of the cerebral cortex are arranged in six distinct layers (Table 29-1).

II. ORGANIZATION

    A. **Projection neurons. Pyramidal neurons** and **stellate projection neurons** either connect one region of the cortex with another or project to subcortical structures.

    B. **Local circuit neurons** inhibit activity within the cortex.

    C. Projection and local circuit neurons are compared in Table 29-2.

Table 29-1
Cytoarchitecture of the Cerebral Cortex

Layers	Name	Contents
I	Molecular	Apical dendrites of pyramidal neurons Local circuit neurons
II	External granular	Small pyramidal neurons Local circuit neurons
III	External pyramidal	Medium and large pyramidal neurons Local circuit neurons Gives rise to corticocortical fibers
IV	Internal granular	Pyramidal neurons Stellate projection neurons Local circuit neurons Receives thalamocortical fibers from VPL and VPM
V	Internal pyramidal	Largest pyramidal neurons; in the motor cortex (area 4) called giant cells of Betz Local circuit neurons Gives rise to corticobulbar, corticospinal, and corticostriatal fibers
VI	Multiform	Pyramidal neurons Local circuit neurons Gives rise to corticothalamic fibers

VPL = ventral posterolateral nucleus of the thalamus; *VPM* = ventral posteromedial nucleus of the thalamus.

III. SELECTED PHOTOMICROGRAPHS

A. Cerebral cortex (Figure 29-1)

B. Alzheimer disease (Figure 29-2)

A

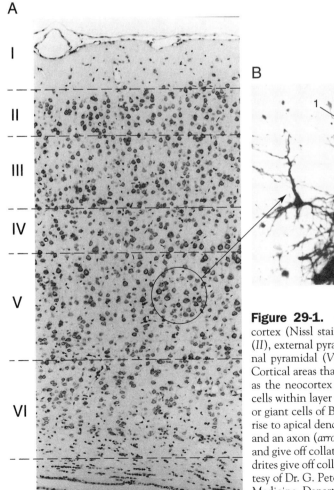

B

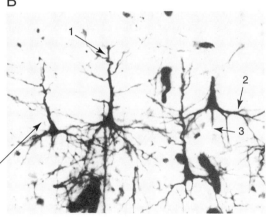

Figure 29-1. (A) A light micrograph of the cerebral cortex (Nissl stain). The molecular (*I*), external granular (*II*), external pyramidal (*III*), internal granular (*IV*), internal pyramidal (*V*), and multiform (*VI*) layers are shown. Cortical areas that contain six layers of cells are referred to as the neocortex or isocortex. (B) A light micrograph of cells within layer V that are called large pyramidal neurons or giant cells of Betz (Golgi stain). Pyramidal neurons give rise to apical dendrites (*arrow 1*), basal dendrites (*arrow 2*), and an axon (*arrow 3*). Apical dendrites often reach layer I and give off collaterals that branch at 90° angles. Basal dendrites give off collaterals that branch at acute angles. (Courtesy of Dr. G. Petersen, East Carolina University, School of Medicine, Department of Anatomy and Cell Biology.)

B. Alzheimer disease (Figure 29-2)

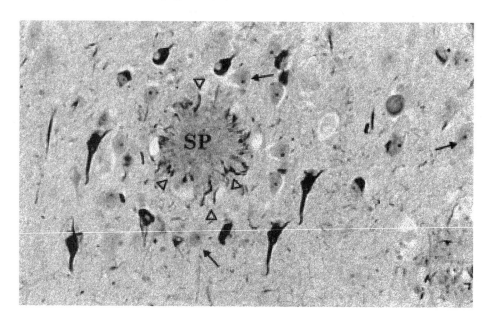

Figure 29-2. Pathologic lesions associated with Alzheimer disease. A senile plaque (*SP*) is shown, which consists of a core of extracellular amyloid surrounded by a halo of dystrophic neurites (*arrowheads*). In addition, a number of dark-staining pyramidal neurons are present due to the neurofibrillary tangles within the cytoplasm. A major component of neurofibrillary tangles is the tau protein, which enhances microtubule assembly. Normal pyramidal neurons are also present (*arrows*). (Reprinted with permission from Siegel GJ, Agranoff BW, Albers RW, et al: *Basic Neurochemistry*, 6th ed. Philadelphia, Lippincott-Raven, 1999, p 951.)

30

Cerebellar Cortex

I. **CYTOARCHITECTURE.** The neurons of the cerebellar cortex are arranged in three distinct layers (Table 30-1, Figure 30-1, Figure 30-2). There are five different types of neurons, including:

   A. **Basket cells** are inhibitory neurons that use gamma-aminobutyric acid (GABA) as a neurotransmitter.

   B. **Stellate cells** are inhibitory neurons that use GABA as a neurotransmitter.

   C. **Purkinje cells** are inhibitory neurons that use GABA as a neurotransmitter.

   D. **Golgi cells** are inhibitory neurons that use GABA as a neurotransmitter.

   E. Granule cells are excitatory neurons that use glutamate as a neurotransmitter.

Table 30-1
Cytoarchitecture of the Cerebellar Cortex

Layers	Name	Contents
I	Molecular	Basket cells
		Stellate cells
		Dendrites of Purkinje cells
		Dendrites of Golgi cells
		Axons of granule cells (parallel fibers)
II	Purkinje	Soma of Purkinje cells
III	Granular	Soma and axons of Golgi cells
		Soma and dendrites of granule cells
		Axons of Purkinje cells convey inhibitory output from the cortex to intracerebellar nuclei
		Cerebellar glomerulus

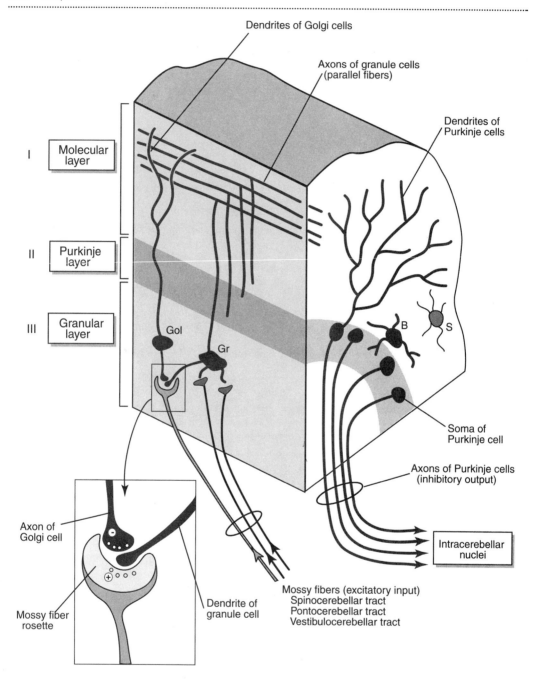

Figure 30-1.   Cytoarchitecture of the three-layered cerebellar cortex. Axons of Purkinje cells, which are inhibitory, are the only output from this region. A cerebellar glomerulus lies within the granular layer (*box*). B = basket cell; *Gol* = Golgi cell; *Gr* = granule cell; *S* = stellate cell; + = excitatory; − = inhibitory.

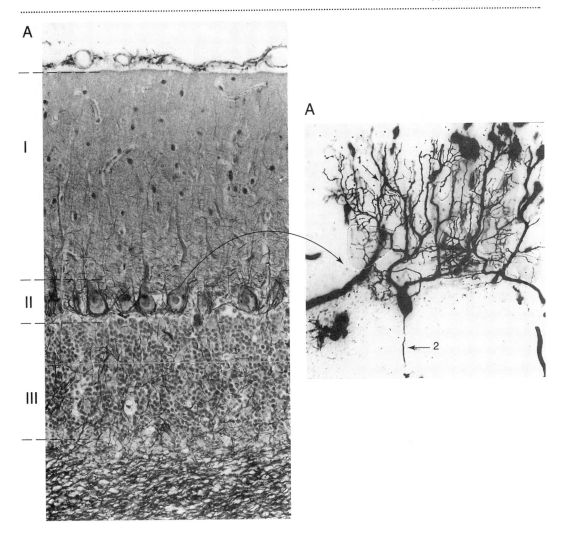

Figure 30-2. (A) A light micrograph of the cerebellar cortex. The molecular (*I*), Purkinje (*II*), and granular (*III*) layers are indicated (silver impregnation). (*B*) A light micrograph of Purkinje cells within layer II. Purkinje cells give rise to an elaborate apical dendritic tree (*arrow 1*) and an axon (*arrow 2*) (Golgi stain). (Courtesy of Dr. G. Petersen, East Carolina University, School of Medicine, Department of Anatomy and Cell Biology.)

II. CEREBELLAR GLOMERULUS (Figure 30-1)

A. **Mossy fiber rosette.** Mossy fibers are axons that synapse with dendrites of granule cells and provide excitatory modulation. They convey excitatory input into the cerebellar cortex from the spinal cord (spinocerebellar tract), pons (pontocerebellar tract), and vestibular system (vestibulocerebellar tract).

B. Dendrites of granule cells

C. **Axons of Golgi cells** synapse on dendrites of granule cells and provide inhibitory modulation.

III. CLINICAL CONSIDERATIONS

A. **Anterior vermis syndrome** results from atrophy of the rostral vermis, which is most commonly caused by alcohol abuse, causing gait, trunk, and leg dystaxia.

B. **Posterior vermis syndrome** results from medulloblastomas or ependymomas that affect the flocculonodular lobe, causing truncal dystaxia.

C. **Medulloblastomas** originate from the granule layer of the cerebellar cortex and usually obstruct passage of cerebrospinal fluid (CSF), causing hydrocephalus.

Index

References in *italics* indicate figures; those followed by "t" denote tables

Glucose, 141t
Glucose-6-phosphatase, 12
α-Glucosidase inhibitors, 127
Glutamate, 55t
Glycine, 54t
Glycogen
    definition of, 12
    liver, 12
    skeletal muscle, 12
Glycogen storage diseases, 12
Glycophorin, 9
Glycoproteins, 25
Goblet cells, 107
Goiter, 152
Golgi cells, 205, *206*, 208
Golgi complex, 3–4, *15*
Golgi hydrolase vesicles, 5
Golgi tendon organs, 45–46
Gonadal hypoplasia, 36
Gonadotrophs, 148t
Gonadotropin-releasing hormone, *170*
Goodpasture disease, *146*
G-protein–linked receptors, 8
Graafian follicle, 167
Granule cells, 205
Granulosa lutein cells, 167
Graves disease, 152, 153t, *154*
Gut-associated lymphatic tissue, 107

Hairy cell leukemia, *92*
Hashimoto thyroiditis, 152, 153t, *154*
Haversian canals, 34
Heart
    blood flow to, 70, 71t
    blood vessels of, 68–69
    circulation to, 70, 71t
    conduction system of, 65, 67
    endothelium, 70
    layers of, 63–65, *64*
Heart block, 67
Heart rate, 67–68
Hematocrit, 78
Hemidesmosome, *21*, 22
Hemodialysis-associated amyloidosis, 29
Hemoglobin, 79
Hemoglobin–oxygen dissociation curve, *80*
Hemolytic anemia, 88
Hemophilia, 86
Hemosiderin, 11–12
Hemosiderosis, 12
Hemostasis, 84–86, *85*
Heparan sulfate, 25
Hepatitis, 119
Hepatitis A, 119
Hepatitis B, 119
Hepatitis C, 119
Hepatitis D, 119
Hepatitis E, 119

Hepatocytes, 116–117, 119t, *120*
Hereditary nephritis (*see* Alport syndrome)
Hereditary nonpolyposis colorectal cancer, 115
Hereditary spherocytosis, 87
Herring bodies, 148
Heterochromatin, 1
High-altitude living, 81
High-density lipoprotein, 116, 117t
Hirschsprung disease, 111
Histamine, 27
Histiocytes, 26–27
Histoplasma capsulatum, 132
Homocystinuria, 28
Howell-Jolly bodies, 87, 101
Howship's lacunae, 34
Huntington disease, 56
Hurler's disease, 6t
Hyaline cartilage model, 34
Hyaline membrane disease, *134–135*
Hyaluronic acid, 25
Hydrochloric acid, 103
Hydrops fetalis, 79
Hydroxyacid oxidase, 5
3-Hydroxy-3-methyglutaryl CoA reductase, 10
17α-Hydroxysteroid dehydrogenase 3 deficiency, 182
Hyperemia, 70
Hypersensitivity reactions, 83–84
Hyperthyroidism, 152, 153t
Hypophyseal portal system, 147
Hypophysis, 147–149
Hypothyroidism, 152, 153t

I-cell disease, 6t
Immotile cilia syndrome, 22
Immunocyte dyscrasias with amyloidosis, 29
Immunoglobulin E antibody receptors, 27, 81
Inhibin, 178, *181*
Inhibiting hormones, 147–148
Inhibitory postsynaptic potential, 52
Inositol 3,4-phosphate, 123
Inositol 3,4,5-phosphate, 123
Inositol triphosphate, 8
Insulin, 123, *124*
Insulin receptor, 123, *125*
Insulin receptor substrate-1, 123
Integrin, 22
Intercalated disk, *50*
Interleukin-1
    description of, *27*
    osteoblast secretion of, 34
Interleukin-6, 27
Intermediate filaments, 6, 7t
Interphase, of cell cycle, 10t
Interstitial cells (*see* Leydig cells)
Intestine (*see* Large intestine; Small intestine)
Inulin, 139, 141t
Ion channel-linked receptors, 8
Iron, 106